PLACING HEALTH

Neighbourhood renewal, health improvement and complexity

Tim Blackman

T0256592

First published in Great Britain in October 2006 by

The Policy Press
University of Bristol
Fourth Floor
Beacon House
Queen's Road
Bristol BS8 1QU
UK

Tel +44 (0)117 331 4054
Fax +44 (0)117 331 4093
e-mail tpp-info@bristol.ac.uk
www.policypress.org.uk

© Tim Blackman 2006

British Library Cataloguing in Publication Data
A catalogue record for this book is available from the British Library.

Library of Congress Cataloging-in-Publication Data
A catalog record for this book has been requested.

ISBN-10 1 86134 610 7 paperback
ISBN-13 978 1 86134 610 0 paperback
ISBN-10 1 86134 611 5 hardcover
ISBN-13 978 1 86134 611 7 hardcover

Tim Blackman is Professor of Sociology and Social Policy and Head of the School of Applied Social Sciences at Durham University. He is a government advisor on health improvement and neighbourhood renewal.

Cover design by Qube Design Associates, Bristol.
Front cover: photograph kindly supplied by Tim Blackman.
Printed and bound by CPI Group (UK) Ltd, Croydon, CR0 4YY

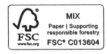

For Julie Blackman 1919–2005

Contents

List of tables and figures

Tables

Figures

Acknowledgements

Many people have contributed wittingly and mostly unwittingly to this book. Thanks must go first to my wife Roberta and daughter Maeve for making such a difference to my life and putting up with my projects. Ideas and comments that have been both influential and challenging have come from, among others, Dave Byrne, Bob Hudson, David Hunter, Linda Marks, Carolyn and Jonathan Roberts, Simon Lewis, Martin Gibbs, Ming Wen, Christopher Hood, Jonathan Wistow, Paul Corrigan and Alan Townsend. Much of the book draws on my experience working as a Neighbourhood Renewal Advisor. I am grateful to colleagues at the Neighbourhood Renewal Unit and in various Government Offices, especially Government Office for the North West and Government Office for the East Midlands, for creating the opportunity to engage with real and difficult issues through this role. Thanks are also due to Middlesbrough Council and the World Health Organization (Europe) for making data available that are used in some of the analyses. I appreciate the support of colleagues in the School of Applied Social Sciences and the Faculty of Social Sciences and Health at Durham University, both administrative and academic, in their efforts to maintain an environment of scholarship and learning that is about making a difference in the world. Finally, The Policy Press has contributed in no small way to this book with their professionalism, patience and attention to detail.

List of abbreviations

ABI	area-based initiative
ADHD	Attention Deficit/Hyperactivity Disorder
BME	black and minority ethnic
BMI	body mass index
CHD	coronary heart disease
CPA	Comprehensive Performance Assessment
CVD	cardiovascular disease
DPH	Director of Public Health
EiC	Excellence in Cities
GCSE	General Certificate of Secondary Education
GDP	Gross Domestic Product
GO	Government Office for an English region
GP	general practitioner
HAZ	Health Action Zone
HIA	Health Impact Assessment
HMR	Housing Market Renewal
IMD	Index of Multiple Deprivation
JAR	Joint Area Review
LAA	Local Area Agreement
LARES	large analysis and review of European housing and health status, a survey undertaken by the World Health Organization (Europe) during 2002/03 in eight European cities
LDP	Local Delivery Plan (of a Primary Care Trust)
LPSA	Local Public Services Agreement
LSP	Local Strategic Partnership
NDC	New Deal for Communities
NHS	National Health Service
NR	neighbourhood renewal
NRF	Neighbourhood Renewal Fund
NRU	Neighbourhood Renewal Unit (from October 2006, part of the Places and Communities Group of the new Department for Communities and Local Government)
ODPM	Office of the Deputy Prime Minister (from May 2006, the Department for Communities and Local Government)
PCT	Primary Care Trust
PPF	Performance Planning Framework

PSA	Public Service Agreement
QCA	Qualitative Comparative Analysis
QOF	Quality and Outcomes Framework
SES	socioeconomic status
SHA	Strategic Health Authority
SLA	service-level agreement
SOA	Super Output Area
SRE	sex and relationships education
VE	virtual environment
WHO	World Health Organization

Preface

To care for places, and to realise the potential of people, are intrinsically good things to do. This book is an investigation of how well we are doing them when it comes to renewing disadvantaged neighbourhoods and reducing preventable causes of illness and death. By renewing neighbourhoods it is possible to tackle inequalities in health that have something to do with where people live. With the arrival in 2001 of England's National Strategy for Neighbourhood Renewal we can investigate whether this possibility is starting to be realised, given that this marked 'a much firmer statement of the desirability of a more spatially equal society than governments have ever voiced before' (Kintrea and Morgan, 2005, p 13). If, as Marmot (2004, p 9) remarks, 'health can be used as a marker of a successful society', then health outcomes across society are both an object of, and a judgement on, such a strategy.

Neighbourhood renewal and tackling health inequalities are interventions in 'wicked problems'; issues that are 'hard to treat' not just because they are complicated but because they are *complex*. In the audit culture of contemporary public policy, the delivery of programmes to tackle these issues is performance managed. This needs to embrace the whole system in which the issues are embedded and assess how far inequality gaps are closing. The major test of these programmes is whether they improve conditions in the most disadvantaged areas at a faster rate than conditions improve for the population as a whole. These challenges of auditing change in whole systems and narrowing gaps as measured by 'floor targets' present a research agenda that currently is catching up with policy innovation rather than leading it.

As chapters in the book argue, complexity theory offers a conceptual framework for making more progress on this research front. The theory is worth serious attention among social scientists and policy makers, and in some quarters is getting it. Complexity is 'out there' as a real phenomenon and there is something extraordinary about the apparent growth of complexity across time as if 'built into the structure of the world' (Gregersen, 2003, p 228). For a while it was Ragin's (2000) book on Qualitative Comparative Analysis (QCA) that gave me a framework for moving on from complexity theory to actual empirical and policy implications, and Ragin remains a big influence. However, in the summer of 2005 I read Robert Wright's book *Nonzero*, which, for me, took the idea of complexity to a new level by arguing that the ongoing elaboration of complexity through biological, cultural and – I would add – policy evolution is a consequence of non-zero-sum dynamics. Wright writes about this on a huge canvas spanning human history and cultures, but I thought about it in relation to the more mundane issues of Local Strategic Partnerships and other recent innovations in English public policy.

I have spent quite a lot of time working with Local Strategic Partnerships and (a) complexity stares you in the face when confronting wicked issues with multiple stakeholders, which is what Local Strategic Partnerships do, and (b) the added value, as hard as it can be to find, arises exactly when the solutions are win-wins. As Wright argues, the effect of (b) is more (a): win-wins drive a further elaboration of complexity. This is inevitable if wicked issues are to be tackled by the cross-sectoral interventions needed where these issues are concentrated most intractably in deprived neighbourhoods. The growing complexity involved in this governed interdependence is challenging the performance management systems that have become such an established feature of public policy in the UK and worldwide. Making performance management work in these circumstances is a current frontier of policy development.

The book has seven chapters. It begins in Chapter One by considering the relationship between health inequality and places, before moving on to introduce recent English policy developments. This then leads to discussing the relative contributions of health care and non-health care interventions, and returns to the issue of places as one of context. The chapter concludes by introducing the concept of a decent neighbourhood.

Chapter Two brings in complexity theory, outlining its key ideas and applying these to thinking about neighbourhoods and their wider environments as open, dynamic and adaptive systems. The chapter establishes a link between complexity theory and Ragin's (2000) QCA method, illustrating this with an original analysis of data on smoking. The chapter then moves on to a broader canvas to consider neighbourhoods as existing in phase spaces, the wider determinants that influence stability and change, with a short case study of Hulme in Manchester. The chapter concludes by discussing the interrelationships of social space and geographical space, identifying the importance of understanding causal combinations as a basis for intervention.

Chapter Three continues the complexity theme by examining the concept of emergence in more detail, linking the complexity concept of an order parameter with the policy concept of upstream interventions in social problems. It considers how complex systems adapt and maladapt, emphasising the importance of a valued future to healthy adaptation. Emergent health problems signal maladaptation, and the chapter considers the example of how alcohol-related morbidity in North West England is threatening to cancel out the recent gains made with closing inequalities in circulatory diseases and cancers. The chapter introduces one of the book's key concepts, environment press, and explores this idea with a novel study of the outdoor participation of people with dementia. The chapter concludes by setting out a causal model of the neighbourhood system.

Chapter Four reviews the evidence for a 'neighbourhood effect' but questions whether such effects can be considered independently rather than in causal combination with emergent outcomes. The role of neighbourhoods in endowing status and self-esteem is considered, along with a discussion of the burgeoning literature on social capital. This leads to a discussion of issues surrounding 'mixed communities' and population mobility. The chapter then considers green neighbourhoods, and the evidence that has been gathering about the apparently substantial health benefits of greenery and nature in the residential environment. It concludes by returning to some of the themes of earlier chapters and with the idea of a decent neighbourhood being a buoying environment.

Chapter Five is a detailed study of the National Strategy for Neighbourhood Renewal, its approach, targets and achievements to date. This chapter gives more consideration to performance management, the governance context of this strategy and public services in England in general. It explores the question of how delivery can be better aligned with good theories and methodologies for closing in on target outcomes, principally those for closing gaps between deprived neighbourhoods and national averages. The chapter then widens its focus to consider the changes in governance represented by innovations such as Local Strategic Partnerships and Local Area Agreements. It concludes by considering lessons learned from evaluating Health Action Zones, principally the need for a dedicated national focus on health inequalities, which is the topic of Chapter Six.

Chapter Six describes recent policy developments in the UK aimed at tackling health inequalities, emphasising particularly the significance of the performance management of delivery. The roles of the National Health Service and local government are discussed, including health impact assessments, and contextualised in terms of the governance developments discussed in Chapter Five. The chapter concludes by returning to consider the neighbourhood as a setting for intervention, but in a wider picture. This is one that includes the growing tensions between targets and performance management on the one hand, and local responsiveness and autonomy on the other. Health inequality sits uneasily within this set of tensions, as it is by definition a commitment to measurement and accountability for performance, but as a wicked issue demands local experimentation and adaptation in order to tackle its many dimensions.

Chapter Seven is about neighbourhoods in this wider picture. It concludes the book by recognising the potential of neighbourhoods as places of engagement, not just with local issues but with the bigger societal landscape. New ways of working and living are emerging locally but in societies of growing complexity. The book ends with some reflections on this emerging, global complexity and the optimistic arguments of Robert Wright (2000) that we are continually learning how to achieve solutions to the challenges that this complexity increasingly poses for social policy and governance.

ONE

Policy and places

This book is concerned with one of the central questions in social policy: what difference does difference make? My main concern in this respect is the difference that places make to people's health. The purpose of this chapter is to introduce the book's framework for exploring this question, set out the policy background, and consider how places matter for health and offer settings for interventions.

People's health in the UK has shown a pattern of steady improvement over several decades. Between 1971 and 2003, life expectancy for males increased from 69.1 years to 76.2 years, and for females from 75.3 to 80.5 years (ONS, 2005a). By 2003, however, there was a gap in estimated life expectancy between professional and unskilled manual social classes of over eight years for males and almost five years for females. Between the best and worst local authority areas the gap was nearly 12 years. Men and women living in the most deprived areas not only live shorter lives than those in more affluent areas, they spend twice as many years in poor health.

It is sometimes argued that the role of local action to tackle health and other social problems is at best marginal to, and at worst a distraction from, the real issues of income and wealth inequality that are the underlying causes of these problems (Pantazis and Gordon, 2000; Ball and Maginn, 2004). The same criticism was made of area-based initiatives (ABIs) to tackle deprivation in the 1970s, a very different era when income inequalities were much narrower than they are now (Community Development Project, 1977). Is it that we have not learned from the 1970s or do places still matter?

Places matter because they are open, dynamic and adaptive systems that do not have a simple cause–effect relationship with national or global drivers of economic, social or policy change. No strategy for tackling health inequalities will reach everyone it should without intervention in neighbourhoods to tackle the local factors that combine with wider determinants of health to create preventable geographical inequalities. This is because there are processes of local emergence at work. These can be investigated empirically but, as with all empirical work, we need a theoretical guide to where to look, what to look for, and what to make of what we see.

An argument of this book is that complexity theory offers this lens. By using complexity theory to understand 'neighbourhoods', we can go beyond the empirical investigation of geographical variation to think about neighbourhoods as complex systems. Neighbourhoods are at the smallest significant socio-spatial scale of the societies of which they are part. They are where population health is an emergent property of interactions on 'home ground' between the levels of the individual and their household, and regional, national and global systems. They are a setting for intervention, but with outcomes more likely to arise from complex causal combinations than linear cause and effect.

Health inequality and places

Little progress had been made with narrowing health inequalities in England by the time the Department of Health first reported in August 2005 on the inequality targets it set out to meet by 2010 (DH, 2005a). This is because there is a long-term trend of widening inequalities in both infant mortality and life expectancy that is proving difficult to turn around. Some important drivers are moving in the right direction, notably falling levels of child poverty, falling levels of sub-standard housing, and falling death rates from circulatory diseases and, to a lesser extent, cancers. It remains a challenge, however, to translate these trends into a narrowing of inequalities given that the most disadvantaged groups and areas need to improve their health at a faster rate than the general improvement that is occurring across the population in general. England is not alone in this respect; there is evidence of a similar long-term trend of inequalities in mortality among other northern European countries (Kunst et al, 2005).

In the UK and many other countries there is a strong relationship between socioeconomic status (SES) and premature mortality, morbidity and disease risk factors. This is particularly true of those diseases that account for most deaths: circulatory diseases (including heart disease and stroke) and cancers. Although deaths from both of these are in decline, they are still concentrated among people with manual or routine jobs and those who are poor or workless.

This social distribution of risk has changed over time. Smoking and obesity are much more prevalent today among people with manual and routine occupational backgrounds than people in professional jobs, but were probably more common among wealthy people in the past (Vågerö and Leinsalu, 2005). In some countries this is still the case. The social distribution of risk also varies geographically. There is, for instance, currently a larger gap between manual and non-manual workers in deaths from circulatory diseases in north-western Europe than in southern Europe.

Within the UK, health varies by country. Results from the 2001 population census enable the proportion of each socioeconomic group self-reporting their health as 'not good' to be compared cross-nationally. There is a similar pattern in all four countries, but the gradient by socioeconomic group is steepest in Northern Ireland, followed by Wales, Scotland and then England (see Figure 1.1). In Northern Ireland, for example, the lowest reported prevalence of 'not good' health is unsurprisingly among higher managerial and professional occupational groups, as in the other countries. At a little over 5%, however, this prevalence is actually higher than among intermediate occupational groups in England. Among routine workers, there is an almost 2.5 times difference between England and Northern Ireland in the proportion reporting their health as 'not good'.

This country effect means that people in the same socioeconomic groups are reporting their health as worse in Northern Ireland than in Wales, worse in Wales than in Scotland, and worse in Scotland than in England. These contrasts are also evident within each country. North

Figure 1.1: General health by country and socioeconomic group, UK, 2001

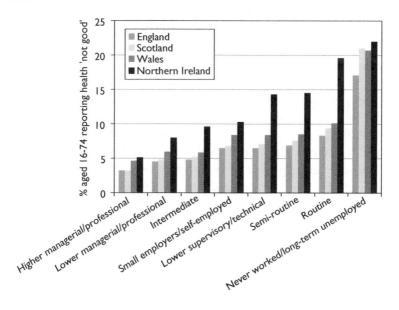

Source: UK Census (2001)

East England, for example, has a similar health gradient to Wales. Overall, this is a different pattern to mortality, which also has a strong socioeconomic gradient but is highest in Scotland, illustrating how the choice of indicator is an important issue if used to allocate resources.

A notable feature of Figure 1.1 is that those with the poorest self-reported health are people who have never worked or who have been unemployed long term. There has been a trend towards the selective exclusion of some people from employment in a number of European countries, much of which is health related. An effect of this is that social inequalities in health are greater across whole adult populations than across only working populations (Leclerc et al, 2006). Worklessness is a distinct dimension of inequalities in health.

There are variations in health on every geographical scale. Data from the World Health Organization's (WHO's) LARES survey enables this to be explored across eight European cities. This survey investigated the effects of housing on health. Here I have used the data to compare the cities on three health indicators: an index of symptoms of cardiovascular disease (CVD) (% with one or more self-reported symptoms); smoking prevalence (% smokers); and a mental health score based on items from the Short Form 36 (SF-36) Health Survey Questionnaire (Bonnefoy et al, 2003). In analysing these data I have restricted cases to individuals aged 18-64 to take into account the effect of age on health, and looked at the prevalence of these indicators by household socioeconomic group. This classification was created by the WHO from a combination of variables regarded as comparable across the cities, resulting in a score that has been categorised into quartiles for the purpose of this analysis. The cities are Angers, France (n=667); Bonn, Germany (n=665); Bratislava, Slovakia (n=733); Budapest, Hungary (n=846); Ferreira, Portugal (n=764); Forli, Italy (n=947); Geneva, Switzerland (n=523); and Vilnius, Lithuania (n=1,460).

Table 1.1 shows the results of this analysis. Ferreira and Vilnius demonstrate the expected gradient of decreasing symptoms with increasing SES score. These gradients are much slighter in Angers, Bonn and Geneva. In Bratislava, Budapest and Forli, there is a threshold effect with high levels of symptoms concentrated in the lowest quartile while other quartiles have similar levels of symptoms. There are also some striking differences between cities in levels of symptoms: the top SES quartile in Ferreira has a higher level of cardiovascular symptoms than the bottom SES quartiles in Angers, Bonn and Geneva. Ferreira also stands out for its very high scores on the mental health indicator, as well as a marked SES gradient. A socioeconomic gradient is also evident in Bonn, but Bratislava, Budapest and Forli again display a threshold effect, with poor mental health concentrated in the bottom SES quartile. Vilnius has high scores in every quartile, with no gradient. Across all the cities, smoking prevalence shows the least variation. In general, smoking prevalence is highest in the bottom SES quartile, but the differences are not great and only reach significance in Angers and Budapest, where there are socioeconomic gradients.

What Table 1.1 demonstrates is the general significance of socioeconomic gradients in health, but also city differences. These are evident in both the steepness of the gradient and a contrast between some cities with a step-by-step gradient and others with a threshold effect. This suggests a city or area effect, and therefore a need to tailor interventions to the nature of the local issue. To achieve the most health gain, the existence of a threshold effect suggests a strategy of

Table 1.1 Relationship between health indicators and socioeconomic group for adults aged 18-64 in eight European cities

| | Household socioeconomic group | | | | |
	Bottom quartile	Third quartile	Second quartile	Top quartile	Significance (chi square)
One or more cardiovascular disease symptoms %					
Angers	11.4	11.4	7.1	8.3	0.499
Bonn	14.3	14.8	15.1	8.4	0.129
Bratislava	25.7	19.6	16.5	15.8	0.447
Budapest	34.9	18.9	19.2	14.6	0.000
Ferreira	40.7	30.4	18.0	15.3	0.000
Forli	25.0	18.6	15.0	10.3	0.072
Geneva	11.9	8.9	7.6	6.6	0.715
Vilnius	23.4	20.7	16.4	13.2	0.018
Poor mental health score %					
Angers	16.1	14.6	10.4	12.3	0.649
Bonn	25.5	20.7	15.1	11.2	0.025
Bratislava	17.1	9.0	12.6	10.0	0.469
Budapest	24.5	14.9	17.4	14.1	0.107
Ferreira	65.4	43.0	33.5	25.0	0.000
Forli	33.3	13.8	11.6	15.8	0.219
Geneva	31.0	24.4	20.4	14.0	0.063
Vilnius	36.6	34.0	27.9	30.2	0.117
Smoker %					
Angers	48.9	37.7	37.8	29.1	0.002
Bonn	42.9	40.9	38.7	30.5	0.117
Bratislava	34.3	29.4	32.0	30.9	0.942
Budapest	49.1	49.1	39.9	32.2	0.003
Ferreira	40.7	29.0	37.1	41.3	0.175
Forli	50.0	40.7	33.3	38.0	0.474
Geneva	48.8	35.6	31.6	38.2	0.213
Vilnius	41.8	43.0	40.4	35.0	0.235

targeting the most disadvantaged group, while step-by-step gradients suggest that general measures across the whole population will be most effective by capturing a much higher number of those at risk (Ashton and Seymour, 1988). However, the latter approach is unlikely to narrow health inequalities unless there are also measures that achieve the most health improvement among those with the worst health.

Above a certain minimum standard of living, social inequalities in themselves may harm health independently of the effect of material deprivation associated with any one socioeconomic group. It has been argued that this works through individual stress arising from the experience of inequality when there are wide *relative* differences in wealth and status (Wilkinson, 1996). Marmot (2004) calls this a 'status syndrome': very unequal societies mean that large numbers of people experience an exclusion from the opportunities, social participation and self-esteem that are enjoyed by some but denied to them. This, it is suggested, causes psychological distress, pessimism or resentment, and increases the likelihood of risky behaviours and illness. It might explain, for example, the statistical link between housing tenure and health that remains even after controlling for social class and income, given that home ownership could be regarded as a marker of status and self-esteem compared to renting (Macintyre, K. et al, 2001).

However, a relationship between subjective social status and health may simply reflect that most people are objectively accurate in assessing their relative social status and the level of material disadvantage associated with it. A longitudinal analysis of Scottish data by Macleod et al (2005) considered both subjective and objective measures of social status and found that subjective status was only weakly associated with mortality once material disadvantage was taken into account. The important determinants of health outcomes appeared to be the father's manual as opposed to non-manual occupation, lack of car access and shorter stature, pointing to the significance of circumstances early in life. They also found that perceived stress increased with higher social position, whether measured objectively or subjectively, but was not associated with poorer physical health. An earlier analysis of the same data found that higher perceived stress was associated with risky health-related behaviours such as more smoking and alcohol consumption (Heslop et al, 2001). But the association of perceived stress with physiological risk such as high cholesterol and blood pressure showed a mixed relationship and appeared to reflect socioeconomic position, with the least advantaged most vulnerable to this effect.

These relationships are not fully understood. Perceived status and stress both appear to matter to health, and indeed might in themselves be regarded as health states in a wider definition of health as well-being. What is clear is that an issue that still dominates health outcomes in a society such as the UK is one of relativities between people's material circumstances.

Minding the gap: from neighbourhood renewal to Spearheads

What is the contribution of *place* to this agenda? We know that people living within the same area often share similar mental and physical states of health. So, targeting services and projects at deprived areas to improve health seems to make sense. But this does not necessarily improve utilisation or change the health-damaging attributes of the areas, and misses people living in deprived circumstances outside the targeted localities. For example, socioeconomic inequalities in oral health remain stubbornly large in the UK, so targeting deprived areas with free fluoride toothpaste is one way of allocating resources to tackle the problem. However, free toothpaste is unlikely to achieve the benefits that follow from water fluoridation, and this need not just be confined to targeted areas. Indeed, to do so would be likely to miss many children living in low-income families.

McLoone (2001) illustrates this issue by showing that if the 20% most deprived postcode sectors in Scotland were targeted for extra resources, only 34% of low-income households would benefit (defining low household income as 40% or more below the national average). Even if 55% of postcode sectors were targeted, accounting for 62% of Scotland's total population, just over a quarter of low-income households would still not be included. In addition, just as 'deprived areas' fail to include many deprived people living outside areas so defined, these areas themselves often have a wide range of incomes, and it is unsafe to assume that an individual is deprived on the basis of their address (McLoone and Ellaway, 1999).

Nevertheless, places cannot be ignored in social policy, because they both concentrate deprivation (and affluence) and have real attributes that affect health and other outcomes. Stafford et al (2001) found from their data on London civil servants that 30% of those in the highest grades compared with only 8% of those in the lowest grades lived in the least deprived wards, while over 40% of those in the lowest grades lived in the most deprived wards. The strong relationship between deprivation and poor health combines with the spatial sorting of local housing markets to create a graded geography of more healthy and less healthy places. Those with the fewest material resources tend to get sorted into the most unhealthy neighbourhoods, even though unhealthy places include people who are neither deprived nor in poor health, just as healthy places include people who are deprived and in poor health. Targeting resources on an area basis will not break the relationship between deprivation and ill–health, but, equally, unhealthy places cannot become more healthy by tackling individual socioeconomic deprivation alone. As well as 'people poverty' or 'people affluence' there is 'place poverty' and 'place affluence' (Powell et al, 2001). The argument of this book, based on the evidence that follows, is that where people live makes a difference to their opportunities for a healthy life.

The existence of 'unhealthy places' is an issue of importance in its own right, a policy object. As long as such places exist in their unhealthy state it is those who are already most at risk of ill-health who are most likely to have little choice but to live in them. Unhealthy places have long been recognised as a danger to wider society because infectious diseases spread (Ambrose et al, 1996). Today, if there are neighbourhoods where immunisation uptake is low then outbreaks of diseases such as measles are more likely because of overall immunisation rates falling below the high level needed across the general population to prevent outbreaks. So what is government policy in the UK doing about health inequalities and the experience of them in *places*?

The current policy position is that these inequalities are not tolerable and in recent years targets have been put in place for narrowing them. This book is mainly concerned with English policy in this respect because since the devolution of policy making in 1998 to the Scottish Parliament and Welsh Assembly there has been a divergence in approaches to how the National Health Service (NHS) is organised, how neighbourhood deprivation and health inequalities are targeted, and how performance is assessed and managed (Mooney and Scott, 2005). But although regeneration and health policies in the countries of the UK have followed rather different paths since devolution, they have all adopted major neighbourhood and health improvement programmes targeted on where conditions are worst. This section of the chapter introduces the English programmes aimed at improving neighbourhoods, reviews the recent emphasis on partnership working, and concludes by considering the general approach to tackling health inequalities.

In England the National Strategy for Neighbourhood Renewal (NR), launched in 2001 as a 10- to 20-year initiative, has the aim that no one should be seriously disadvantaged by where they live because of 'failing' local services or a poor environment (SEU, 2001). There is also a range of related initiatives that have a neighbourhood focus, such as New Deal for Communities (NDC), Sure Start programmes and their successor children's centres, extended 'community' schools, Neighbourhood Management, and the Safer Stronger Communities Fund, which is aimed at tackling antisocial behaviour, drugs, crime and improving the condition of streets and public spaces. The Housing Market Renewal (HMR) initiative is also part of the picture, and a response to some of the perceived failures of past urban policies that were seen as too locally focused (ODPM, 2003a). HMR is aimed at restructuring housing provision at a conurbation or sub-regional scale to create more mixed-income neighbourhoods, including demolition and redevelopment in some of the poorest areas of England where 'neighbourhood sustainability' is seen as the key challenge.

Funding for NR programmes was initially allocated to the 88 most deprived local authority areas in England. Allocations were made with the expectation that the growing mainstream budgets for public services would get behind the local NR strategies and that there would be further targeting of the most deprived neighbourhoods within each local authority area. The focus is on closing gaps between national averages for life expectancy, the employment rate, educational achievement, crime and decent housing (with liveability added subsequently) and these local authorities' averages, as well as between targeted neighbourhoods within the local authority areas and their local authority averages. The current health inequality targets are:

Reduce early deaths (under 75) by 2010:
- from heart disease and stroke so there is a 40% reduction in the gap between the national average and the poorest areas; and
- from cancer, with a reduction in the inequalities gap of 6%.

Reduce the health gap between the poorest areas and the national average by 10% as measured by infant deaths under age one and life expectancy at birth.

Tackle the underlying problems of ill-health and inequalities by 2010 by:
- reducing adult smoking rates to 21% or less with a reduction to 26% or less for routine or manual groups; and
- reducing the under-18 pregnancy rate by 50% with faster progress in the most deprived wards (NRU, 2005a, p 5).

The local delivery vehicles for the National Strategy for NR are Local Strategic Partnerships (LSPs), one of the most important innovations in local governance in recent years. These bring together the local authority, the local NHS, other public bodies, community groups and business representation, and have now been established in every local authority area of England. In the NR areas they have a key role in planning, funding and monitoring delivery to meet the NR targets. Although there is freedom in how NR LSPs deploy their funding allocations, regionally based Government Offices (GOs) are responsible for assessing their performance and can intervene or suspend allocations if it is judged unsatisfactory.

Another way of losing funding is to succeed in meeting targets. Within a few years of the NR programme starting, six NR areas were judged by 2005 to have made enough progress for their NR funding to be phased out. Yet, at the same time, a new issue came into focus: small pockets of deprivation, including but extending beyond NR areas, and leading to the Safer Stronger Communities Fund being introduced in 2006. This focuses resources on these small localities in 84 local authority areas. The new focus was enabled by technical advances in the official Indices of Deprivation used to measure geographical disadvantage and allocate funding. Pockets of deprivation previously masked by the more affluent areas surrounding them have been picked out by the improved spatial detail offered by developments in data technologies.

There is considerable emphasis on 'mainstreaming' what works from the NR strategy and related initiatives so that successful new ways of working become part of normal practice in how public services are organised and delivered. There is strong political pressure to demonstrate results from the higher spending as soon as possible, despite the long-term perspective heralded as new when the strategy was launched. An obstacle to making faster progress is commonly regarded to be a lack of flexibility about new ways of working and poor targeting, coordination and community engagement. This is often summarised as a failure to 'join up'.

In theory, LSPs are where things get joined up strategically at the level of local governance. Although local authorities and NHS organisations locally have a swathe of targets that their individual services are expected to meet, it is through LSPs that some of these targets are shared across these and other organisations. In the NR areas, these include the targets for reducing inequalities in health, worklessness, crime and poor housing, and improving education and liveability. Although some LSPs have run into problems with bringing different interests together in a way that adds value compared with working outside the LSP structure, they are becoming established as an emerging new system of local governance. LSPs are partnership bodies, but it is increasingly recognised that the local authority, as the directly elected local public body, should be 'first among equals' in leading their work (Lyons, 2006).

In every local authority area in England, LSPs now have a key role in developing and delivering Local Area Agreements (LAAs). These are plans that are agreed between local organisations, predominantly the local public sector, and national government. They are designed to improve the targeting of resources, remove duplication and achieve critical mass in budgets that are not in organisational silos but organised to tackle cross-cutting issues. The main agenda in this respect are the 'wicked issues' that Rittel and Webber (1973) identified over three decades ago as the most difficult to tackle because there is less certainty about the problem and less agreement about the solution than 'tame' problems that are well defined and have clearly right or wrong solutions.

Health inequalities are a prime example of a wicked issue and are being addressed in the development of shared targets in many LAAs. England's health inequalities strategy, launched by the *Programme for Action* in July 2003, set out ambitious targets to be shared across government departments and agencies (DH, 2003). This sharing of targets was an innovation designed to achieve partnership working and joint accountability. There were similar target-setting health inequality initiatives in Wales and Scotland, but not as yet the same degree of performance assessment (Greer, 2006). The *Programme for Action* set out plans for meeting national targets for reducing socioeconomic gaps in infant mortality and geographical gaps in life expectancy, shared with the NR strategy. Over a period of a few years, health inequalities moved from firstly being recognised as a policy issue, to then being framed as targets to be met, to now being a key outcome for which the NHS is held responsible, sitting alongside reducing waiting times, tackling hospital-acquired infection and expanding patient choice as one of its six main priorities (DH, 2006a).

This responsibility is shared with local government and LSPs but the recent focus on the role of NHS services in reducing health inequalities reflects a concern that progress has been too slow to meet the national targets by 2010. By focusing on identifying those who are already ill or at risk due to problems such as smoking or obesity, and targeting treatment accordingly, it is expected that more progress can be made in the short term than interventions in the wider determinants of health that have a longer-term payback period. Tackling wider determinants such as child poverty and poor housing remain priorities, and the *Programme for Action* extended a requirement for health impact assessments of new policy proposals from all government departments. This wider focus received significant support from the final Wanless Report on the future of the NHS, which urged greater progress with improving public health and reducing health inequalities in order to avoid escalating treatment costs (Wanless, 2002).

Related to these developments, local government and the NHS are seeing the neighbourhood dimension of their work more strongly emphasised. The Department of Health is basing 'a sustained realignment of the whole health and social care system' on 'community well-being' (DH, 2006b, p 19). More services will be delivered in settings closer to people's homes, with the NHS and local government commissioning services informed by feedback from users and surveys, and expected to join up as a 'whole local system' (p 20). This reorientation is being paralleled by changes in local governance that are framing the 'neighbourhood' as an organisational level for service delivery and coordination, performance management and partnership working, and a scale for involving the public in decisions. It is not yet clear at what scale this new level of devolution might be, although population sizes of 5,000-10,000 are mooted. New powers are being proposed at this level for parish or community councils to deal with antisocial behaviour, for residents to trigger action by public services in response to persistent problems, for allocating community funds for residents to spend on neighbourhood priorities, and for local residents to run and own assets such as community centres and recreational facilities (ODPM/Home Office, 2005). The devolution of health care commissioning to primary care organisations offers further opportunities for community councils to be involved in decisions about local health care services (DH, 2006b).

Localism is very much on the governance agenda in England. However, neither the NR strategy nor the *Programme for Action* is solely concerned with geographical inequality and 'place poverty'. The *Programme for Action* addresses differences between socioeconomic groups as well as between geographical areas. All NHS Primary Care Trusts (PCTs), which are the bodies in England responsible for governance of the local health care system, are expected to include in their plans measures for tackling local inequalities in health, whether or not they are in a deprived local authority area. The fifth of local authority areas with the worst health and deprivation indicators are expected to make faster progress to meet the national targets, and the 88 PCTs in these areas, the so-called Spearhead Group, are receiving additional resources to help meet their inequalities targets. (At the time of writing, PCTs are undergoing a restructuring, which will reduce their number and, in all but a few, align their boundaries with unitary or county councils, give them a stronger strategic role and see detailed commissioning of health care services pass to primary care practices.)

The Spearhead Group of PCTs leads the NHS push on deprivation-related ill-health in the targeted local authority areas, which include around 28% of the national population (DH, 2005b). Other initiatives include the national network of over 250 Healthy Living Centres; a Healthy Schools programme prioritising achievement of 'healthy schools status' for 7,500 schools serving deprived catchments; 25 Communities for Health pilot areas for community-based health improvement work; the Healthier Communities Programme involving 12 local authorities in demonstration projects to tackle health inequalities; the Beacon Council scheme, which has seen four local authorities awarded special status for their work on tackling health inequalities and disseminating results to other local authorities; and the Race for Health programme to deliver race equality through language initiatives.

The current health inequality targets are nationally framed in the sense that Spearhead PCTs are expected to close the gap between their areas as a group – the worst 20% – and the England average. There are no national Spearhead targets for closing gaps *within* these areas, although local NR strategies are expected to formulate these for their localities, including for health. There is, furthermore, a debate about whether differences between the health of areas and groups should be measured in relative or absolute terms, with the current English targets a mix of the two (Low and Low, 2006). Absolute differences appear to be a very direct way of measuring whether progress is being made, but it is possible for an absolute difference to decline while a relative difference remains unchanged. Low and Low (2006) point out that the current cancer target of achieving a 20% reduction in premature mortality across the board, and a 6% reduction in the absolute gap between the England average and the Spearhead districts, actually implies the Spearhead Group improving more slowly than the average! This is of course the opposite of the policy intent. While it might be argued that it is the intent that is important, as I return to in the concluding chapter, these targets matter if there is to be wider public engagement with them as an issue of the relativities that are acceptable in a society.

There is also an issue with the types of inequality targeted. Mental health and ethnic inequalities in health are two important examples. South Asians, for instance, are 40% more likely than the rest of the population to contract coronary heart disease (CHD) and around 50% more likely to die prematurely from it, but there are no targets to close these gaps (DH, 2005a). There is a well-established link between mental health problems and deprivation, as well as variations by ethnic group. Part of the reason for these gaps is poor data availability when the strategies are strongly based on measurement. Ethnic monitoring is improving but is still often very patchy and data on mental health are very limited in both scope and availability. Black and minority ethnic (BME) communities are defined as only broad groups by the population census, yet some of their health risks need more specific targeting that is sensitive to behaviours and beliefs that will affect the acceptability and success of interventions. Another dimension of inequality neglected by recent ABIs is urban and rural differences. Levin and Leyland (2006), for example, show how Scotland's rising health inequality between deprived and affluent areas has been highest in remote rural Scotland, while Halliday and Asthana (2005) argue that there was an urban bias even in the predominantly rural Health Action Zone (HAZ) they studied.

Urban areas are of course easier to target, but the map of deprivation at any scale and on virtually any measure is dominated by urban areas, despite the importance of access and transport in areas with more scattered settlements. Local authorities and their PCTs were included in the Spearhead Group if they were in the worst fifth for at least three out of five selected indicators. Four of these are health indicators and one uses the Index of Multiple Deprivation (IMD), which includes an access component. The effect of the IMD being only one of five indicators is that the Spearhead Group is not the same as the NR areas, which are based on the worst-scoring areas on only the IMD measures. There is a substantial overlap, as would be expected, but nine Spearhead local authorities receive no NR allocations, while 24 NR areas are not in the Spearhead Group (DH, 2005a; ODPM, 2005a). The two strategies, therefore, are not entirely joined up and have slightly different health inequality targets.

Places and access to health care

To what extent are the health inequalities targeted by these programmes about inequalities in access to care and treatment or inequalities in income, housing or other wider determinants of health?

Although the UK has a universal publicly funded health care system, this has not eliminated geographical variations in the health of the public. The NHS may even contribute to these inequalities despite its funding locally being weighted to reflect the pattern of ill-health, based on premature mortality. Although there is a tendency for general practitioners (GPs) to gravitate towards more affluent areas, in recent years there has been a drive in the NHS to achieve universal prompt access to GP services, and to modernise primary care premises in deprived areas (NHS Modernisation Board, 2004). The centrepiece of the latter is the £1 billion LIFT programme that has refurbished and replaced hundreds of GP and community nursing premises, often as part of a broader regeneration scheme that has included incorporating services such as local authority 'one-stop shops' for advice and information, fitness amenities and community cafes in the new buildings (NAO, 2005). But it remains the case that there are fewer GPs and practice staff per head in deprived localities, and in some areas, notably London, there are still GP practices that are single-handed or lack a practice nurse. Reaching primary care and hospital services can also be a problem in rural areas and in deprived areas where there is low car ownership (Hamer, 2004).

Whether this actually means that access to health care is worse in deprived areas is not known with any certainty. In Canada, a country also with a universal health care system, a significant difference in the use of GP services has been found depending on travel/visit time (Law et al, 2005). A UK study based in Northamptonshire found that both transport availability and distance affected access to GP services, but the relationships were complex (Field and Briggs, 2001). Many of those at the greatest distance from surgeries had better access to a car, and the most severe access difficulties were often encountered at intermediate distances of four to five miles where a high proportion of patients were dependent on public transport.

A recent analysis suggests that in one English region, the North East, geographical proximity to general practices is greater than elsewhere in more deprived areas, despite most PCTs in the region having fewer GPs per head than the national average (Adams and White, 2005). This study used the IMD 2000 for electoral wards in North East England (average population just over 5,000) to compare the IMD's 'access domain' with the employment, education and income domains of the index. The access domain is a combined measure of average straight-line distance to the nearest general practice, post office, food shop and primary school. The authors carried out their analysis separately for urban and rural wards. A significant correlation was found between the access domain and the socioeconomic deprivation domains, suggesting that those wards with greater deprivation tended to have closer geographical proximity to general practices. This was true of both urban and rural areas, with the correlation being stronger for rural wards despite common assumptions that access is an issue in these areas.

Adams and White's findings contradict Tudor Hart's (1971) famous 'inverse care law', which would predict poorer access to primary care in deprived areas. But there are a number of limitations to the study, as the authors acknowledge, including using an access indicator that combines four local services and is not specific to just primary care. This measure also does not indicate either the quality of primary care available or actual utilisation, and the study is confined to North East England. A further qualification is that, while the correlation coefficients reported are statistically significant, they leave much of the variation in local access unexplained. For example, even the highest negative correlation reported between rural wards' rank on the access domain and rank on the income domain, -0.58, means that only 34% of the variation in access reflects variation in deprivation. In urban wards, where most people live, only 7% of the variation in access is explained by deprivation, despite statistical significance at the $p=0.01$ level. This is encouraging from an equity viewpoint but does not mean that deprived areas are necessarily well served in relation to their health needs.

The validity of the access domain of the IMD is taken up by Niggebrugge et al (2005). They compare the IMD 2000 access scores for electoral wards in East Anglia with a range of more detailed indicators of travel times and bus availability for visiting a GP. A relatively low correlation was found, especially for rural wards, indicating that the IMD access domain is not a particularly good measure of local access to primary care. The authors point out that the access domain is largely based on the local population in receipt of benefit payments, and therefore may not reflect accessibility for the local population as a whole. This will also affect Adams and White's (2005) conclusion in that it would be expected that wards with higher levels of deprivation will have more deprived people living close to GP services, especially as deprivation is associated with higher-density urban areas. For deprived people as a whole, including those spread more thinly across a larger number of, on average, less deprived wards, access may not be as good as Adams and White suggest.

There is quite a striking variation in the number of GPs per 100,000 weighted population across England's PCTs, with a range from 40.6 to 83.5 shown by data for 2005 (DH, 2006c). And it is the PCT areas with the poorest health outcomes that have the fewest GPs. This issue is targeted for action by the recent community services White Paper, and PCTs will be expected to commission additional primary care services for under-served areas, including the option of using social enterprises or private companies to increase primary care provision (DH, 2006c). It remains the case, however, that whether this variation in GP coverage has an impact on health status or health inequalities is unclear (Reeves and Baker, 2004). Beyond the UK, this 'inverse care law' can be a serious contributor to health inequalities where there is not a publicly funded universal health care system. A prime example in the developed world is the US, where variations by metropolitan area in the supply of primary care physicians mean that whether an area is well served or poorly served is reflected in mortality rates (Shi and Starfield, 2001).

This might suggest that within the UK the different levels of spending by country on the NHS will be reflected in health outcomes. NHS expenditure per capita in 2002/03 was, compared to England, 16% higher in Scotland, 12% higher in Northern Ireland and 9% higher in Wales. These higher levels of expenditure are in fact not reflected in better population health or even higher levels of public satisfaction with NHS health care (Alvarez-Rosete et al, 2005). They are also not reflected in higher levels of activity, such as outpatient and inpatient cases, and waiting times were lowest in England, where the strong target-led approach to performance managing waiting times has contrasted with the other countries. Overall, these comparisons imply that how resources are deployed and how factors outside the NHS system influence health are more important to health outcomes than levels of spending, certainly within the range of expenditure per head represented across the countries of the UK.

Within the NHS, these issues of how resources are deployed and accessed include, for instance, how patients from disadvantaged backgrounds are treated by receptionists and doctors, as well as the attitudes of many poor people that their health problems are simply due to getting old, even if they are still in their fifties or sixties, and therefore not worth going to the doctor about. Documented examples of these inequalities in access and use of health care include GPs spending less time in consultations with more deprived patients, fewer consultations about preventative health care among people from social classes IV and V compared with I and II, and fewer hip replacements among people from lower socioeconomic groups (Farrington-Douglas and Allen, 2005).

Ethnic inequalities in access are a further issue. For example, there is a lower take-up of cancer screening and immunisations among BME groups. One of the factors that contributes to this is fewer female GPs in areas with high concentrations of Asian residents, and the effect of this on women taking up cervical cancer screening. Thus, as well as geographical coverage, the issue of unequal access to effective health care interventions includes considering how both patients' and health care professionals' backgrounds, attitudes and aspirations can create obstacles to presenting with symptoms and accessing effective treatments.

The neighbourhood is an important scale at which to consider and act on these issues. Older people and low-income families without a car are less able to travel easily to where services are, and are more likely to need services to come to them or be grouped together locally. Matching provision to need, however, is about actual use and not just distance. Increased budgetary and professional flexibilities in the NHS and local government are creating a capability to reconfigure services to improve utilisation by reflecting patterns of need and choice both geographically and socially. This ranges from a PCT's power to contract with a diversity of possible service providers, to wider public health roles for groups such as community pharmacists and environmental health officers. In the London borough of Barking and Dagenham, for example, a simple decision to let pharmacists run the PCT's needle exchange scheme resulted in a 200% increase in use (Cole, 2003). Outreach is especially important: a recent innovation is health trainers, recruited locally in deprived areas to engage people individually with the personal support needed to improve their health. For the general population, new NHS Walk-in Centres are a similar example of health care provision reaching out to where people lead their lives, whether as residents, shoppers, commuters or visitors (DH, 2004a).

Health care is often argued to be a relatively unimportant influence on health status compared to the contributions of low income or poor working and living conditions to *causing* health problems. This view receives much support from the substantial evidence of strong associations between SES, environmental conditions and health (Acheson, 1998). However, taking heart attacks as an example, while having a manual working background has been found to have a very marked effect on increasing the risk of a heart attack, it also decreases the chance of reaching hospital alive *and* the probability of surviving a month after an attack (Macintyre, K. et al, 2001). The inverse care law is probably part of the explanation for this social class effect but is only the last stage in a chain of risks that extends back to events during gestation and in infancy, with their major health effects several decades later (Power at al, 1996). There is, though, still uncertainty about the contribution that broad public health interventions can make to reducing health inequalities, and it has been suggested that these become relatively less important than health care interventions as populations become more affluent (Craig et al, 2006). I return to this issue later; at this stage I want to return to the fact that affluence is certainly not a condition shared universally in the UK.

The power of context

MacDonald and Marsh (2005) found in their study of young people growing up in the depressed areas of Teesside that most *chose* to remain living in very deprived neighbourhoods, despite poor job prospects and widespread problems with crime and drugs. Close, local family networks were the most important reason for this, but it also seems that these neighbourhoods were widely regarded as 'normal', rather than excluded or disadvantaged, because neighbourhood deprivation was so extensive. Local social divisions were perceived instead at a very fine-grained scale, such as streets or parts of an estate with troublesome residents or blighted by vacant houses or criminal activity.

MacDonald and Marsh, however, are writing about the families that stayed in these areas. The more unequal a society, the more likely people are to move away from neighbours who are poorer than they are and into neighbourhoods with more status, where homes are a sounder investment, the environment is cleaner, greener and safer, and schools are popular. Area effects are both a cause and an outcome of these individual strategies.

Individual strategies are played out on landscapes structured by market forces and public policies that create greater or lesser inequality (Byrne, 1999). For neighbourhoods to decline there need to be conditions that make leaving the neighbourhood possible: jobs and homes that are qualitatively better and within reach. As I discuss in the next chapter, growing affluence can threaten to deepen the marginalisation of many deprived neighbourhoods because new choices present themselves for at least some of their residents. The human preference to be with similar others, which MacDonald and Marsh argue puts a break on their young people wanting to move to a 'better' neighbourhood, can fuel geographical divides when individual circumstances improve. Individual decisions to move house may actually have surprisingly extreme aggregate effects, especially when tolerance of difference is low and there is the space to do something about it.

We can make a first use of complexity theory at this point to understand how this might happen. Batty (2005) uses the complexity concept of 'emergence' to model how extreme patterns of segregation can arise from the self-organised behaviour of individual agents, behaviour which at an individual level would not seem extreme. He considers two types of model. The first is where individuals change their opinion depending on change in the presence of other individuals with a differing opinion in their local neighbourhood. The second is where individuals change their location with respect to the presence of other individuals with differing opinions or attributes in their neighbourhood.

The first model begins at a random starting point and a threshold rule is applied for when an individual changes their opinion or behaviour, depending on whether this is shared by a neighbouring majority or minority. When the model is run over time, a chain reaction occurs that leads to a steady state of dramatically segregated clusters of similar individuals. Disturbing this state by changing the distribution of individuals results in a return to a highly segregated pattern. In the second model, a grid system of cells is used whereby individuals do not change their opinion but move from one cell to another to avoid neighbourhoods where they would be in a minority. The resulting degree of segregation depends on the availability of empty cells (the availability of choice) and the level of tolerance to difference. A significant finding of this model is that levels of segregation emerge that are much greater than individuals' own tolerance of different individuals would suggest. Overall, and based on the assumptions used, the models show that where individuals are content up to a point to live with other individuals with different characteristics, but are not content to be in a minority, striking and surprisingly high patterns of segregation emerge. Only a few discontented individuals are needed to trigger an unravelling that leads to these highly segregated distributions.

Batty does not explore the policy implications of his models in any depth but clearly, if these simulations do reflect real behaviour, they suggest two conclusions of policy significance. The first is that the extent of choice is a key parameter: the more choice there is, the more individuals segregate themselves, and to a degree that goes beyond what their individual preferences would predict due to the effect of positive feedback. This implies that current New Labour policies in the UK of expanding choice in the public services and in spheres such as health care, housing and schools sit awkwardly with policies to narrow inequalities. Given that a degree of segregation between neighbourhoods may emerge from individual choices that is greater than individuals would themselves choose for their society, then there is a case for intervention to limit the extent of segregation as a *societal* choice.

The second conclusion that could follow from Batty's modelling is that tolerance of difference matters, and this too is a key parameter. A more tolerant society is less likely to be segregated, with the implication that 'mixed communities', for example, are unlikely to be sustainable if people have a low level of toleration of difference. This again can probably be influenced by public policy, such as programmes to promote community cohesion. But it is also plausible that if inequalities are wide and obvious then individuals are less likely to tolerate differences with their neighbours. They will either do something about it (such as move out of the neighbourhood) or experience dissatisfaction and possible health consequences, along the lines argued by Marmot (2004). It is interesting in this respect to note that the evidence of a link between the degree of income inequality and local population health is much weaker at small spatial scales than for whole regions or countries, possibly because social contrasts are more obvious at these larger scales (Drukker et al, 2004).

The attributes of a neighbourhood, and how different it is to other neighbourhoods, matter to some people more than others. For instance, people who are less mobile are likely to spend more time in their home area and be more dependent on local services. However, as mobility has increased with growing car ownership, and as housing choice has widened with the spread of owner-occupation, there is evidence that more people are choosing where they live and commuting to work (Dorling and Rees, 2003). This is fuelling a continuous process of spatial filtering. In the UK, the effect of this when combined with the persistence of marked income and wealth inequalities has, certainly over the period between 1971 and 2001, been one of continued socio-spatial polarisation, and 'areas now more easily than ever typified as being old and young, settled and migrant, black and white, or rich and poor' (Dorling and Rees, 2003, p 1287).

Burrows et al (2005) add the phenomenon of internet-based neighbourhood information systems (IBNIS) to this increased capacity, for those who are able to do so, to choose their neighbourhoods to reflect the qualities they want for themselves and their children. The website <www.upmystreet.co.uk> is an example, available to those with access to the internet to check the social profile of neighbourhoods at postcode level, as well as the value of property, the level of crime and the examination results of local schools. These websites avoid offensive terminology given that their advertising is often aimed at achieving commercial sales across a range of income groups. But it is clear that easy access to ACORN© descriptions such as 'well-off workers, home owning family areas' and 'multi-ethnic, severe unemployment, lone parents' is 'likely to contribute to ongoing processes of inter-neighbourhood segregation and intra-neighbourhood homogenisation' (Burrows at al, 2005, p 55).

Batty's two models of segregation processes chime with the distinction often made in research on area health effects between compositional effects and contextual effects. Compositional effects are about who our neighbours are, and how health and health-related attitudes and behaviours are influenced by the overall socioeconomic make-up of the neighbourhood. Contextual effects are about the sort of place somewhere is in terms of its environmental features, such as crime or air quality, which impinge directly on individuals' states of health and may also affect their health-related behaviour, such as smoking more, walking less or leaving altogether a neighbourhood perceived to be unsafe. Both are thought to contribute to 'neighbourhood effects' that impact on individuals' health in addition to, and often in combination with, their individual characteristics and household circumstances. Popay et al (2003) find them both reflected in people's accounts of what makes 'good' and 'bad' neighbourhoods, although with a third dimension being apparent: a sense of belonging and pride in the neighbourhood. Compositional effects are echoed in notions of 'community spirit', respect for others and for property and trusting others, while contextual effects are reflected in notions of safe streets, clean environments, trees, play areas, youth facilities and convenient shops and public transport.

Neighbourhoods, therefore, are combinations of attributes of the environment and the people living there. These interact so that, for example, the neighbourhood can reflect on ourselves and our sense of identity and status. This can mean that the effect of income inequality on health may be different depending on the neighbourhood. We saw evidence of this kind in terms of the city effect on the relationship between SES and health revealed by the LARES data. Another dataset that I can use to illustrate this point is from a town-wide residents survey conducted in Middlesbrough, in North East England, in 2003. The data include respondents' self-reports of their health as 'good', 'fair' or 'not good', and their incomes in one of three weekly income groups of under £200, £200–£249 and £250 or higher. The analysis was restricted to 18- to 64-year-olds.

In the relatively affluent neighbourhood of Nunthorpe, the proportion of residents in the lowest income group of under £200 a week reporting their health as 'not good' was 35%. This is very similar to the lowest income group in one of Middlesbrough's very deprived neighbourhoods, North Ormesby, where the proportion was 34%. But in Nunthorpe, increased income is associated with improved self-reported health: the proportion reporting their health as 'not good' declines to 19% in the middle income group and then to 14% in the upper income group. In North Ormesby, increased income appears to make little difference to self-reported health. The proportions reporting their health as 'not good' are 34% among the middle income group and 30% among the upper income group. Being poor appears to affect health to a similar extent whether someone lives in affluent Nunthorpe or deprived North Ormesby. However, this is not the case at higher levels of income: this seems to offer little benefit to health in North Ormesby, suggesting that the living environment may be so bad as to work against the potential health gain of higher incomes.

Even the most evidence-based, well-funded and effectively delivered health interventions may fail to achieve sustainable improvements if there are features of the neighbourhood that mean there is not a receptive context. These problems can include poor access to primary care services locally, sub-standard housing, poor employment opportunities or high levels of crime. Social capital, too, is increasingly recognised as a factor (see Chapter Four). This point about the power of context is a specific instance of the general approach of realistic policy evaluation, which models interventions as 'mechanisms' using the formulation: context + new mechanism = outcome pattern (Pawson and Tilley, 1997). People in places are bounded contexts, which have a possibly determining influence on how and whether a new mechanism 'works'.

Because poor health tends to cluster geographically, neighbourhoods are seen as part of the solution to tackling health inequalities. Neighbourhoods differ along dimensions that appear to be very significant for health: environmental stress and availability of local social support, infrastructure such as shops with affordable healthy food or safe parks; transport connections and the accessibility and availability of health services; and prevailing attitudes in the community towards health and health-related behaviours such as exercise and smoking. Vertical and horizontal 'joining up' are novel if still often elusive features of the programmes targeted on neighbourhood deprivation and their intended impact on mainstream services. Shared strategic, managerial and financial responsibility between PCTs and local authorities is growing, how budgets are spent is becoming more flexible, partnership working is expected to extend beyond the main public bodies to voluntary and community groups, and local and central government have formally adopted 'shared priorities' that include tackling health inequalities.

Overall, these developments mark a shift to a concern with *outcomes* rather than any fixed pattern of provision. Indeed, patterns of provision have become fluid, with restructures and new initiatives creating a frequently changing landscape. Amid this fluidity in organisational systems, neighbourhoods offer some continuity of focus. The qualities of the surroundings in which we live are among the main concerns about quality of life that are reported in surveys of residents in the UK (MORI, 2002). Places matter, and as more than the administrative partitioning of space to implement policy: they are where abstract strategy is concretised.

Places are also where knowledge is concretised and where it is possible to learn about 'what works'. Outside the bounds of place and time, knowledge is abstract and at best an averaging across many local contexts. While this can reveal common patterns and relationships, it risks losing knowledge of what actually happens and works in specific places. It is still possible to arrive at general understandings of causes and outcomes, and these may point to underlying structures and processes that operate over large spatial and temporal scales, but their effects can be different from person to person, place to place and time to time. In the language of realistic evaluation, 'what works' depends on where, when and with whom an intervention is implemented (Pawson and Tilley, 1997). The outcomes are rarely simple but occur as patterns. There is, in other words, always an interaction with context.

Time as much as place forms this context. There are lags of sometimes many years between implementing measures to improve health and seeing the health outcome pattern emerge. For many effects, time cannot be simply played back by reversing an effect by the same amount that it increased forwards. This is illustrated in a study by Sacker et al (2006) of how individuals who leave employment with a limiting illness often do so in response to a limited job market, but they may not move back into employment until there has been a considerable rise in labour demand well beyond that when they left their job.

Neighbourhoods are more than just a context. They are open systems and what happens in a neighbourhood is affected by other systems. Work pressure, for example, can affect people's level of neighbourhood social participation, while having no work can compound the exclusion experienced by living in a deprived area. These effects are mixed up in the real world so we should be very cautious about separating them for analytical or intervention purposes. Individual effects are not placeless but interact with places such as through processes of spatial sorting and segregation, and through different individual vulnerabilities to adverse neighbourhood conditions. Individuals' health is also affected by who they live with – their household system – and an increasing number of studies have highlighted a strong household effect on health (Chandola et al, 2005; Sacker et al, 2006).

Indeed, this clustering of health at the household level, due to factors such as shared consumption, behaviours and housing conditions, may partly explain *area* variations in health, which should therefore be considered as emergent from a combination of contextual, compositional and household risk factors. Health does not seem reducible either to person or place but to arise from time- and place-contingent causal combinations. This seems to be why Shouls et al (1996) find that health inequalities between affluent and poor individuals are greater in less deprived areas, or Sundquist et al (2006) find that the incidence of CHD shows a strong association with a measure of social capital based on neighbourhood differences in voting turnout. The whole system needs to be considered, but this has to be framed in a way that allows for intervention. The neighbourhood is one such framing. For example, damp houses are likely to affect the health of their occupants, and some more than others, but it makes little sense to invest resources in eradicating damp from the properties affected if crime is so high in the neighbourhood that residents take every opportunity to move out. Residents are unlikely to want to stay because their respiratory health is better but their mental health is still compromised by such a stressful living environment.

Decent homes and decent neighbourhoods

Home inside the front door, and whether it is damp, cold, noisy or overcrowded, sits within the wider neighbourhood context of which it is part, and which together exercise place influences on people's health. The health effects of dwellings and neighbourhoods are often considered separately in research studies and policy documents (Barrow and Bachan, 1997; Battersby et al, 2002; Thomson et al, 2002; British Medical Association, 2003). Housing, however, is *experienced* as the dwelling *and* its residential setting, the neighbourhood. Hazards such as burglary, noise or lead in drinking water, and psychosocial aspects such as the ontological security of 'home ground' and social status, are

Table 1.2: Effects of housing and neighbourhoods on health

	Direct effects	Indirect effects	
		Individual/household level	Area/ neighbourhood level
Physical/ material attributes	Damp, cold, mould, heat, homelessness	Indicator of social and economic status	Services and facilities; features of the natural and built environments
Social/ meaningful attributes	Rent/mortgage arrears and in/security of tenure	Household and area culture and behaviours	
	Feeling of 'home', social status, ontological security	Reachability of services and facilities	Neighbourliness, community safety

Source: Adapted from World Health Organization (Europe), 2004.

features of both a dwelling and its neighbourhood. Table 1.2 summarises the factors involved.

In the mid-1980s, about 9% of the English housing stock was assessed as 'unfit for human habitation', a definition based on disrepair, the adequacy of facilities for preparing and cooking food, and dampness. By 2001, a new official housing quality indicator based on a set of criteria for a 'decent home' resulted in 33% of the housing stock being judged as failing this standard (ODPM, 2003b). There has not been a dramatic decline in housing quality but a change in the standards used, notably the inclusion of thermal comfort. Nevertheless, the period of 20 years between 1981 and 2001 appears to have been one of a widening gap between the quality of housing and people's *expectations*, a key factor in understanding how many neighbourhoods, especially in old post-industrial areas, are experiencing low demand and in some cases abandonment (Kintrea and Morgan, 2005).

The decent homes standard is not explicitly based on health criteria but its constituent elements are clearly relevant to health: whether the dwelling is weatherproof, in disrepair, in need of kitchen or bathroom modernisation, or provides sufficient thermal comfort (ODPM, 2004). Whether the link has been broken between poor individual health status and living in conditions likely to be damaging to health can be considered by looking at the proportions of well and unwell people living in decent or non-decent housing. The 2001 English House Condition Survey (EHCS) shows that 36.5% of people reporting a limiting long-term illness or disability lived in non-decent housing, compared to 32.5% in the general population (ODPM, 2003b). The proportion of people with a limiting long-term illness living in non-decent housing is likely to decline significantly if the government achieves its target for England of all social housing meeting the decent homes standard by 2010. However, this excludes many people in poor health who do not live in social housing. They are unlikely to see the same progress with improved housing conditions, given that for the private sector there is only a more general commitment to reducing the proportion of 'vulnerable' (benefit-dependent) households living in non-decent conditions. A more comprehensive target has been ruled out as unaffordable, an issue that applies equally to extending the target to neighbourhoods.

In contrast to decent homes, there is no official definition of a decent neighbourhood in the UK, although the English House Condition Survey adopted a measure for 'poor neighbourhoods'. This is based on a neighbourhood having over 10% of its dwellings assessed as seriously defective or other serious environmental problems. In 2001 11% of the national housing stock was in 'poor neighbourhoods' based on this measure (ODPM, 2003b). Although the data are not directly comparable, Kintrea and Morgan (2005) estimate that this represents an increase from 6.6% in 1996. While substantial progress was made over this period with reducing the proportion of non-decent housing (from 46 to 33%) the opposite appears to have happened with non-decent neighbourhoods, at least until 2001.

This trend is also discernible from surveys by the market research company MORI, and other local surveys, which have been reporting for several years that large numbers of residents are concerned about local crime and antisocial behaviour, dirty streets, neglected spaces and lighting, and the lack of facilities for young people (MORI, 2002). These issues are often among the most important improvements to public services that residents want to see. Residents' assessments of the 'visual quality' of their local area are also very important in determining whether they are satisfied with their neighbourhood in general. When combined as an index along with two other measures of 'physical capital' – the prevalence of flats over five storeys high and terraced houses – these assessments have been shown to explain statistically two thirds of the total variation in residents' satisfaction with their area (Collinge et al, 2005). This is a larger effect than deprivation, widely regarded as the main influence on how satisfied people are with their neighbourhood and local services. It seems, too, from a study by Parkes and Kearns (2006), that antisocial behaviour and fear of crime affect residents' health, the latter more consistently than the direct experience of crime. This study also found that a better appearance of the neighbourhood was consistently associated with better health, controlling for other factors.

MORI survey data show that between 1988 and 2003 respondents' satisfaction with their general standard of living rose, but satisfaction with their residential area as a place to live declined (Page, 2003). Surveys of residents' satisfaction with local government services have also revealed sharply declining overall satisfaction, despite real increases in local spending, and perceptions of poor liveability appear to have been partly behind this trend (Lorimer, 2004). Since 2003, however, there is evidence of these perceptions of neighbourhood liveability improving, including in some of the most deprived areas, although the gap with other areas remains large (Collinge et al, 2005).

This improvement has coincided with liveability rising up the political and spending agendas of central and local government. New legislation and a range of initiatives in recent years have been aimed at enhancing local councils' powers and resources to improve and maintain neighbourhood environments and control antisocial behaviour (Hastings et al, 2005). Many councils are improving their performance with better and more responsive environmental services and schemes such as community wardens. This progress has been driven by initiatives at the centre of government, notably the Liveability Team in the Office of the Deputy Prime Minister (ODPM) (reorganised as the Department for Communities and Local Government in May 2006) and the Anti-Social Behaviour Unit in the Home Office, as well as the appointment of a Minister of Communities and Local Government. Major regeneration programmes such as NR and NDC are also beginning to have an impact on neighbourhood environments. A tracking between 1999 and 2003 of 12 low-income areas with renewal programmes by Paskell and Power (2005) revealed that the number of problems originally identified as blighting the neighbourhoods dropped by a third over this period, a scale of change that is 'visible and significant' (p 48), although some areas were not turning around, and the authors emphasise that a continuing long-term commitment is needed in all the areas.

These are significant developments for public health. Neighbourhood liveability has important implications for mental health, physical health and health-related behaviours such as smoking and exercise. Neighbourhoods, therefore, are settings for health interventions, but are not empty vessels waiting to be filled with 'health projects'.

Conclusion: places in context

It is well established that health in certain places is worse than in others, but this is about more than geographical variation. Geographical differences in health are patterned by processes that sort people between different types of place habitus. For Bourdieu (1977), habitus is fundamentally about class habitus and the forces of class structuring that advantage some and disadvantage others. Those with the resources to do so can advantage themselves by living in cleaner, greener and safer neighbourhoods.

There is more to this than liveability. Class is important in both the Marxist sense of command over economic resources and the Weberian sense of market position and associated prestige and status. Health inequalities deriving from command over economic resources 'might be incorporated into personality in the form of locus-of-control' while those deriving from prestige and status 'might be incorporated into the personality in the form of self-esteem' (Scambler, 2002, p 94). Neighbourhoods are where we feel more or less in control of the surroundings in which we live, and more or less buoyed by the status of where we live. This matters to our health, but neighbourhoods are not just background environments. They are people–environment systems, and we can use complexity theory to explore what this means for health as a neighbourhood phenomenon.

TWO

Health, neighbourhoods and complexity

An introduction to complexity theory

This book argues that improving health in neighbourhoods can be informed by using complexity theory. The reason is that neighbourhoods and their 'states' are outcomes of complex causation.

A relationship whereby A causes B in a linear and mechanical fashion is simple (echoing the last chapter's point about 'tame' problems). Many such relationships operating together is complicated. *Complexity* arises when there is *interaction* between many elements, such as the relationship between A and B depending on interactions with C, D or E (a 'wicked issue' in policy terms). When this happens, emergent and difficult-to-predict properties can arise from the interactions.

While traditional quantitative research in the social sciences is concerned with analysing relationships between variables, such as the relationship between income inequality and rates of premature mortality, complexity theory focuses on *cases* as empirical and actual domains. The interest is in the 'states' of these cases; not so much how and why variables change but how and why cases change. There is a direct concern with context in this respect, which variables-oriented quantitative research tends to regard as a difficulty to be controlled for, rather than part of explanations. The nature of cases as configurations of compositional and contextual attributes that combine to produce emergent outcomes can be described and investigated in either qualitative or quantitative terms (Byrne, 2002).

Cases, whether individuals, households, neighbourhoods, organisations or economies, are conceptualised within this theoretical framework as complex adaptive systems with self-organising behaviour. They are open to their environment and therefore affected by it, and have characteristics that are often fuzzy, not least their boundaries. Fuzzy in this context means that cases are not necessarily crisply defined in terms of having or not having key attributes (key attributes being those that are causally linked with outcomes of interest). A case may be in one attribute category say 80% and in another say 30% (Ragin, 2000). Examples of neighbourhood attributes in this respect could be segregated/mixed, safe/unsafe or green/barren. The important thing about the extent of 'in or outness' is its causal significance in terms of changes in state.

Whether complexity theory is useful depends on whether the world is one of interactions, emergent properties and non-linear changes. There does appear to be plenty of evidence that this is the case, although it is an empirical question (Eve et al, 1997; Byrne, 1998; Cilliers, 1998; Wright, 2000; Gregerson, 2003; Meen et al, 2005). In terms of health and place, phenomena such as the 'epidemiological transition' and 'area effects' are non-linear and emergent. The former describes the qualitative transition in the state of population health that occurred in developed countries as their main causes of mortality changed from infectious diseases to degenerative diseases such an CHD and cancer. Among many examples of area effects is Meen et al's (2005) demonstration of non-linear effects in how deprivation thresholds trigger movements into and out of local areas. They show that it is only when deprivation falls to a certain point that housing market demand begins to take off.

Complexity is evident in the interconnectedness and interactions that characterise neighbourhoods and urban systems, organisations and disease processes in general (Sweeney and Griffiths, 2002; Stacey, 2003; Batty, 2005). In terms of the desired added value from partnership working, complexity also describes the 'emergent property' of more joined-up and successful policy and interventions that should arise from interactions between organisations on, for example, an LSP. Chapter One noted a policy recognition of complexity in attempts to join up programmes and share priorities across agencies through LSPs and LAAs in order to tackle 'wicked issues'.

Wicked issues are problems whose causation is complex because of interdependencies, with solutions that are not clear and require collaboration across a range of services (Clarke and Stewart, 1997). Chapter One also demonstrated complexity in how different local contexts affect how a relational property such as socioeconomic inequalities in health has different expressions in different places, and how interventions are likely to be affected in a similar way. The principle of complex emergence was mentioned on a number of occasions and illustrated directly with Batty's models of segregation. Neighbourhoods, the chapter argued, are open, dynamic systems nested within other systems, with inputs and outputs and emergent properties such as health and liveability.

Complexity and neighbourhood systems

Luhmann (1995) argues that social systems exist in an environment of other systems from which they are differentiated by being 'self-referential'. This means that systems achieve, through the communication of information, relations with themselves and a differentiation of these relations from relations with their wider environment. Complex systems are, however, open systems and interact with their environment, often making it difficult to define their boundaries. The position of the observer will often determine how these boundaries are defined, such as whether that observer is a local resident or a statistician, and therefore the purpose of describing a system defines how it is 'framed' (Cilliers, 1998).

Neighbourhood boundaries may be created administratively, by defining political or service delivery boundaries, or statistically using a technique such as cluster analysis to create spatial classifications that minimise within-area variation and maximise between-area variation. These two approaches can also be combined to create 'natural' neighbourhoods for the purposes of local governance or resource allocation, perhaps modified by local knowledge about community boundaries. Experientially, however, the neighbourhood starts as we leave our front door. Where it ends varies according to many spatial and temporal factors but, in public health terms, the concept of a walkable zone of experience is important.

People endow a neighbourhood with organisation through their walking patterns from the nodal points of their homes – walking children to school, walking to the bus stop or local shops, and walking to call on neighbours. This behaviour, however, is also structured by the locations of schools and shops, physical boundaries such as roads, and housing markets such as different tenures and associated socioeconomic boundaries. Neighbourhoods are embedded in housing markets, travel-to-work areas, political units, built environments and the areas served by schools, hospitals and other services. They are constructed by these wider systems in a top-down way but they are also instances of bottom-up emergence from local, self-referential interaction. To a greater or lesser extent, most people feel surrounded by a neighbourhood, their residential surroundings. But the extent to which a neighbourhood emerges empirically depends on whether local interactions create collective variables – common attributes – that are to some degree geographically shared and bounded as group properties.

Neighbourhoods are bounded configurations of attributes, but these configurations interweave with the attributes of other systems, such as the individual, their household or the local labour market. So the framing of a neighbourhood does not mean that all the interactions present in a neighbourhood are occurring at the same scale. We can regard key attributes beyond the neighbourhood scale as parameters, while key attributes at the neighbourhood scale can be regarded as collective variables, such as liveability. For most people, and certainly for people on low incomes and groups such as children and older people, the experience of these collective variables is likely to concern quite a small geographical area or 'home ground' within five to 10 minutes' walk from home (Stafford et al, 2003). This is a meaningful, spatially limited and proximal system in which the environmental experience is important. Of particular significance is that the qualities of this home ground signify status. A 'good neighbourhood' is not only one where people want to live but also one where saying you live there means something positive about yourself and who you are.

Where a bad neighbourhood ends and a good one starts is one aspect of the difficulty of defining system boundaries. There may be a clear and obvious boundary but it is also a question of perception; one person's good neighbourhood may be someone else's bad. People's sense of belonging to a neighbourhood and their perception of its boundaries and qualities depend on who they are as well as where they are: their lifestyle, mobility, length of residence, age, income or disability, for example.

So, understanding and intervening in neighbourhoods needs a perspective that is at multiple scales. For instance, it is possible to work upwards to the economic environment in which the neighbourhood is located or downwards to households and individuals. Time is also an essential part of the approach, because all these systems are on trajectories through time. If a transformation occurs in one system this can affect another system and possibly transform it as well. Some examples are considered in this chapter; what complexity theory aims to do is to link these levels to produce coherent explanatory accounts of change.

Complexity and neighbourhood renewal

Renewing neighbourhoods to narrow health inequalities is not a mechanical procedure because rarely are there relationships of the type A causes B. The issues exist in a 'zone of complexity' where interactions introduce uncertainty and agreement needs to be negotiated between multiple players (Stacey, 2003).

It is, however, possible to understand some of this complexity at a level of reasonable detail. This can be achieved by treating the neighbourhood as a clustering of attributes with causal implications for outcomes. Fontaine and Gourlet's (1997) work on fatal road traffic accidents shows how these accidents are emergent outcomes of combinations of type of person, type of road and time of day. Using the statistical technique of correspondence analysis, they identified four clusters: older pedestrians crossing a road in urban areas, child accidents in urban areas during the daytime while playing or running, intoxicated pedestrians involved in night-time accidents in the country whilst walking on the road, and pedestrians involved in secondary accidents and changes of transport mode. The place combination of these attributes at certain points of time produced a risk landscape in space and time. In complexity theory such phenomena are known as attractors. Fontaine and Gourlet draw the conclusion that the most effective way to reduce fatal accidents is to design interventions that remove these attractors.

The scale of the challenge facing England's NR strategy is of course very different to customising accident prevention measures. Turning round such a range of targets across so many localities is a very ambitious goal. For a start, it is difficult for neighbourhood-focused programmes to meet objectives like reducing worklessness because key upstream drivers are beyond the neighbourhood scale. These are known as order or control parameters in complexity theory and the demand for labour is an example. While neighbourhood programmes such as customised training for inward investors or providing business premises have some impact, they are downstream interventions that may be necessary but not sufficient to reduce worklessness.

The economic system includes parameters that fundamentally affect neighbourhoods. But a neighbourhood's own 'state' is a crucial factor in considering its sustainability within a given set of economic conditions. There is now a focus in urban policy on what makes a neighbourhood 'vulnerable', and the answer lies in how a neighbourhood's state combines with its environment. Green et al (2005) conceptualise the key features of a neighbourhood state as community assets or *capitals* that produce a flow of services or *benefits* for local residents. Four capitals are identified: fixed capital in housing, plant, roads and so on; human capital in the form of residents' levels of education, skills and health; environmental capital, or the amenity of the neighbourhood; and social capital and levels of trust and respect in the neighbourhood. The decline or successful renewal of neighbourhoods depends on these capitals, but in interaction with wider control parameters: especially those of sub-regional housing and labour markets.

Qualitative change in local conditions is an indication that change in one or more control parameters has fundamentally affected the local system. A control parameter, however, can be internally produced by collective action within the system as well as be external to the system. In both cases the effect is on collective variables that change to produce a qualitative transition in the system so that it is different to what it was before. Kelso (1995, p 45) comments:

> Collective variables and control parameters are the yin and yang of the entire approach, separate but intimately related. You don't really know you have a control parameter unless its variation causes qualitative change; qualitative change is necessary to identify collective variables unambiguously.

This is not a determinist model. There is no one-to-one relation between a parameter value and the coordinative patterns generated by a system's behaviour. This behaviour is also not just affected by control parameters but also by general fluctuations, which may introduce instabilities sufficient to bring about a state transition if positive feedback starts to occur.

Nevin et al (2001) help to clarify this with their work on the risk of neighbourhood abandonment in the North West of England. They operationalised neighbourhoods as clusters of adjacent enumeration districts (units of several hundred people) with similar housing and social characteristics. They found that conditions internal to the neighbourhood that increased the risk of abandonment were high concentrations of economically inactive, unemployed and retired people (that is, the attribute of worklessness) *combined with* high concentrations of privately owned terraced housing or social rented housing with concentrations of flats (the attribute of housing form). The key external factors were the level of employment and the interest rate, as these influenced how many people could exit from unpopular residential areas through finding employment and being able to buy a property elsewhere.

Concentrated worklessness is a necessary condition for low demand but Nevin et al suggest that it is not sufficient on its own to bring about abandonment. A sufficient combination of conditions arises when there are 'obsolescent' housing forms and a wider economic environment conducive to house purchase outside areas of low demand. Better opportunities for employment and house purchase pose the main threat to 'at-risk' deprived neighbourhoods rather than increasing deprivation. When decline occurs it is non-linear, with vacancy rates reaching a critical point and then, in the absence of intervention, vacancies becoming entrenched in a positive feedback process driven by the effects of stigma and dereliction on the supply of new residents (Lee and Nevin, 2003). The same type of process is identified by Ormerod (1997) in explaining the wide spatial variability in crime rates, and the rapid rise in crime that can occur in some neighbourhoods as a threshold point is passed.

Both national economic and policy systems include control parameters that fundamentally affect the circumstances and futures of neighbourhoods. These parameters, such as an interest rate, can also respond to bottom-up signals from lots of local systems. For instance, England's Sustainable Communities Plan is aimed at tackling both neighbourhood decline in the North and the Midlands, and the opposite problem of housing shortages in the South East of England, and emerged from local problems with low housing demand in some localities and housing shortages in others (ODPM, 2003a). The NR strategy, conceived on the basis of a rather different philosophy of renewing rather than replacing neighbourhoods, and engaging local people in local solutions, was not seen as sufficiently regional in scope to tackle the scale of urban restructuring thought necessary to tackle these low-demand problems (Lee and Nevin, 2003). The result was a new high-level policy system, the Housing Market Renewal (HMR) initiative. The designation of sub-regions of low housing demand spanning local authority boundaries followed, with intervention in their property markets including extensive compulsory purchase, demolition and large-scale, long-term investment in new multi-tenure housing. The strategy is not only a response to significant spatial concentrations of low house prices and vacant homes, which had been features of many old industrial areas for a number of years, but to the speed at which neighbourhoods were abandoned in the late 1990s.

A high-level system acts across groups of lower-level systems but in interaction with them. This interaction includes the possibility of transformation in the state of either the lower or higher order system (or both). For example, the HMR initiative has in places been contradicted by a recovery in some local property markets, substantially increasing the cost of intervention, but also challenging the rationale for intervention. Protests by residents who do not want to be displaced by redevelopment have followed in a number of places. This type of phenomenon – interaction between higher- and lower-level systems – is what Kelso (1995, p 9) describes as the 'circularly causal underpinnings of pattern formation in nonequilibrium systems'. It gives complexity theory what Williams (1999) regards as a feature of realist theory in general and that is 'ontological depth', rather than simply horizontal cause–effect chains of explanation.

Collective variables give a system the group properties or attributes that enable it to be defined, such as the housing and social characteristics used by Lee and Nevin (2003) to cluster enumeration districts, and the turnover and void rates used to identify neighbourhoods at risk, on the margins of risk or not at risk of a non-linear process of decline. Other collective variables define higher-level systems such as labour markets. Some of these collective variables – the ones of greatest interest in research and policy terms – are order parameters that govern a system's behaviour. There is, however, a great deal of contingency in this respect because some order parameters may only operate to cause fundamental change when they reach critical values and combine with other parameters. For example, a parameter such as the local employment rate may only operate as a cause of neighbourhood in-/out-migration when configuring with some other attribute such as neighbourhood liveability.

Although it may theoretically be possible to determine what will happen a neighbourhood as a result of these interactions if all the relevant variables are known and can be modelled, in reality this is never likely to be achievable. This is why statistical modelling of relationships between variables rarely accounts for more than half of the variation in the outcome variable. Furthermore, very similar systems (in terms of their attributes) can have different states (in terms of an outcome). Similarly, different systems may occupy the same, common state. Not all deprived areas of social housing, for example, present high risks of child accidents, even though there is a general relationship between the two attributes. Attributes may be necessary but not sufficient to produce an outcome; they may need to be in combination with one or more other attributes to have an effect. In policy terms this implies not only that intervention in certain key conditions may achieve significant change in an outcome, but also that there may be signatures or fingerprints that can be detected in advance of upcoming change, offering the prospect of preventative intervention. But unless a condition is of such causal significance as to be sufficient on its own to cause an outcome, attention always needs to be paid to local interactions and how these introduce contingency into causal processes.

Ragin (2000) accepts this 'messy' nature of reality with his method of Qualitative Comparative Analysis (QCA), but causal explanations are still regarded as possible. In QCA, different configurations of attributes are investigated for how they are associated with an outcome. Thus, the same configuration of attributes across many cases may result in different outcomes, while different configurations may be associated with the same outcome. Some attributes, which might be regarded as order parameters, may be sufficient on their own, regardless of any combination with other attributes, to produce the outcome.

A worked example: the complex causation of smoking

Smoking has a sharp socioeconomic gradient and contributes substantially to the much higher incidence of premature deaths from cancer and circulatory disease the greater the level of socioeconomic disadvantage. Regular smokers who die from a smoking-related disease lose on average 16 years of life expectancy compared to non-smokers (Walrond et al, 2004). The NHS runs smoking cessation services, using nicotine replacement and bupropion, which are very cost-effective but are making little headway with reducing smoking prevalence among deprived communities (Milne, 2005). The higher rate of smoking cessation among less deprived groups means that the socioeconomic gap in smoking and related morbidity and mortality is set to continue widening.

There is an as yet largely unexplored area which might be called the ecology of smoking that could offer a targeted approach to reducing the socioeconomic gap in smoking rates. A statistical association between neighbourhood-level deprivation and smoking has been demonstrated by several studies (Kleinschmidt et al, 1995; Reijneveld, 1998; Duncan et al, 1999; Ross, 2000; Shohaimi et al, 2003). While there appears to be a neighbourhood deprivation effect on smoking that is independent of whether an individual is deprived or not, less is known about the particular features of local environments that could be behind this relationship. Both the neighbourhood rate of non-employment and low levels of social participation and trust (or 'social capital') have been identified as candidates (Lindström, 2003; Öhlander et al, 2006). Psychosocial conditions in the workplace may also have an effect, either directly through job strain or indirectly by reducing social participation.

Pickett et al (2002) consider the role of social context on health-related behaviours generally, in terms of whether this context is present oriented or future oriented. A context of deprivation may mean hopes for the future are low. Combined with a lack of resources to do anything about deprivation individually, preventive health behaviours that are future oriented are likely to receive a low priority compared to coping with more immediate stressors. Smoking can bring relief and pleasure in the here and now. If resources are limited in conditions of adversity, they are more likely to be deployed for short-term survival than to make stage-setting moves that invest in the future (Chisholm and Burbank, 2001).

I have explored these issues by analysing data available from Middlesbrough Council following their household interview survey in 2003. Middlesbrough has a population of around 140,000 and is one of the most deprived local authority areas in the UK. Data are available from the survey for a representative sample of 7,351 adults. Removing respondents living in wealthier areas to reduce possible confounding and including income in the analysis, which had a lower response rate than other questions, reduced the sample size to 2,882. Still representative of the population of Middlesbrough's less affluent neighbourhoods, the data provided an opportunity to undertake a cross-sectional analysis of a range of factors that could be associated with smoking. Worklessness, low income, a low level of education, neighbourhood problems (liveability) and unhelpful neighbours were selected as indicators of the type of limited resources and adverse circumstances that could encourage smoking and discourage cessation.

Worklessness is the condition of being either unemployed or out of the labour force and not retired or in full-time education. These states are effectively indistinguishable when looking at the probabilities of a transition to employment and at health status, notably poor mental health (Goldsmith et al, 1995). The evidence suggests that the direction of causation from worklessness to illness is greater than the inverse, but this is a complex issue (Mclean et al, 2005). As a causal factor, worklessness is likely to damage a person's locus of control as well as representing a loss of social role, with health effects that are about more than just the income deprivation associated with being out of work (Marmot, 2004). In the Middlesbrough sample, smoking rates among respondents who were retired, in full-time education or employed were in the range 24.6% to 30%, while rates among those who were looking after home and family, caring for a sick or disabled person, unable to work due to long-term sickness or unemployed were in the range 57.7% to 67.7%. A dichotomised variable of workless/ not workless was computed for the analysis.

Liveability was conceptualised in terms of resident perceptions of visible neighbourhood disorder or neglect. How the neighbourhood looks reflects on how much we feel in control of how it looks, and how we believe others see us. This introduces the potential for dissonance between where we live and where we would want to live, with risks of stress and possible health damage (Popay et al, 2003). An index of visible neighbourhood problems was computed based on whether any of derelict land and buildings, empty houses, fly-tipping or litter were 'serious concerns', and whether any of the following needed improving 'a lot': green spaces, children's play areas, street lighting, repairs to the roads and pavements, and the condition of housing. Responses were summed for each respondent by scoring each report of a serious concern or needing a lot of improvement as '1' to give a cumulative score for a 'liveability' variable. The frequency distribution of the scores was graphed and this showed them grouping into three categories of 0 (high liveability), 1-2 (moderate liveability) and 3 or more reported problems (low liveability). The average smoking prevalence in the lowest category was 25.6%, in the middle category 32.1%, and in the highest category 40.4%.

Two variables to measure the social environment of the respondent's perceived neighbourhood were also included. The first was based on answers to the question of whether neighbours were willing to help each other out, dichotomised between strongly agree/agree and disagree/strongly disagree/don't know. Smoking prevalence among the first group was 31.6%, rising to 40.8% among the second group. The second measure was whether the respondent had experienced a burglary in the past year. Smoking prevalence among respondents who had been burgled was much higher than among those who had not, at 54.5% compared to 32.9%.

Net weekly income was categorised into three groups based on breaks in the frequency distribution: £250 plus, £200-£249 and less than £200. Smoking prevalence across these three income bands was 23.9%, 31.3% and 38.6% respectively.

The questionnaire asked about respondents' level of education, classifying this as higher education, further education, or no education beyond the minimum school-leaving age. Education adds a dimension beyond income of individual status. It is unlikely to be a direct contributor to smoking behaviour because the risks of smoking are widely known, and a large majority of smokers report that they want to quit, with little variation by socioeconomic group (Lader and Meltzer, 2003). Non-smoking norms in high- and medium-status circles and the subjective experience of low prestige encouraging compensating comfort behaviour such as smoking may be relevant factors (Bartley, 2004). Levels of smoking were 18.7% for those with higher education, 27.5% for those with further education, and 37.5% for those with no further or higher education.

There was no significant difference by gender in the sample, but this variable was included in the multivariable modelling to explore its effect. There was also no clear pattern by age except for a noticeable decline in smoking among respondents aged 65 or older. Smoking prevalence was 35.6% among those under 65 compared to 24.6% among those aged 65 plus. This partly reflects the national pattern in that older age groups are much more likely to have stopped smoking, often because of their health problems. Ethnicity was included in the analysis given the known variation of smoking rates by ethnic group (DH, 2000a), although Middlesbrough's BME population, which is largely of Pakistani origin, is small and made up only 7.5% of the sample. Similarly, mental health status was included, based on respondents reporting whether or not they 'have experienced mental health difficulties'.

As the respondent's neighbourhood was based on their perception of their local residential environment rather than a pre-defined area, it was not possible to use multi-level analysis, and the number of cases in any given neighbourhood beyond the large administrative area of an electoral ward would also have precluded this approach. Instead, logistic regression and QCA were used. All except one of the variables selected for analysis demonstrated significant bivariate associations with smoking. The one exception was gender, which did not show a bivariate relationship with smoking but was significant in a multivariable logistic regression model, and improved model fit sufficiently to justify inclusion.

Following a number of iterations, a final logistic regression model was derived. The independent effect of each variable, controlling for the effects of the other variables, is summarised as follows. Being workless had a significant effect on increasing the likelihood of smoking, with an odds ratio of 2.71 (2.13-3.45). Education had a significant effect, with some evidence of a dose–response relationship. The odds ratio for smoking of further education compared to higher education was 1.68 (1.33-2.13), and that of no further or higher education compared to higher education was 2.46 (1.77-3.42). Income and liveability showed a similar relationship. Both burglary (1.88, 1.20-2.96) and unhelpful neighbours (1.50, 1.23-1.84) increased the odds of smoking, as did white ethnicity (3.47, 2.35-5.12), reporting mental health difficulties (2.09, 1.43-3.04), being aged under 65 (2.01, 1.57-2.59), and being male (1.32, 1.11-1.57).

Logistic regression is a variable-based rather than case-based method. While the technique has confirmed theoretical ideas about what are likely to be important factors that influence smoking behaviour, in the real world these factors are unlikely to be independent of each other but to occur in causal combinations. Focusing on cases rather than variables enables these combinations to be investigated.

QCA can be used to explore how cases cluster into groups that are qualitatively different in outcome, defined by different configurations of attributes. It is based on selecting attributes relevant to an outcome of interest and then exploring every possible combination of them to examine what cases fall into each combination and with what outcome. The technique is an alternative to logistic regression or multi-level modelling in that QCA does not seek to isolate independent effects but to understand outcomes as associated with multiple configurations of conditions. This is a better representation of the real world, where people live with conditions such as worklessness, age, ethnicity and neighbourhood problems that are 'mixed up' rather than experienced as separate independent effects (Macintyre and Ellaway, 2003; Oakes, 2004).

Ragin's fsQCA software was used to carry out a case-based analysis with those variables used for the logistic regression that represent conditions of limited resources or environmental threats in people's lives: worklessness, poor liveability, low education, unhelpful neighbours and low income. Burglary was excluded because of low prevalence (3.1%). The analysis uses categorical variables dichotomised between the 'worst' category (for example low liveability) and the 'not worst' categories (for example moderate or high liveability). Other analyses not reported here were carried out with more variables and using all categories. These revealed some interesting patterns but often with a small number of cases in the configurations and a lack of statistical significance.

Table 2.1 shows the 18 configurations with more than 30 cases, accounting for 2,617 of the 2,780 cases included in the analysis. Smaller configurations are excluded because of the unreliability of calculating proportions from such small numbers. The first configuration in the table has the highest smoking prevalence, 74.5%. Along with the three other configurations that exceed a smoking rate of 50%, it includes worklessness. The fifth highest smoking rate configuration of 46.5% does not include worklessness, but has every other condition associated with smoking present. Thus, either worklessness on its own in any combination, or all four of the other conditions being present, are associated with very high rates of smoking, and might be regarded as 'sufficient' conditions in this respect. Then what occurs in the table is a pattern of smoking rates declining as the conditions associated with smoking decline in number, so that the lowest rates are where only one or two conditions are present, and the very lowest rate of 10.3% has all conditions absent. There is, however, one exception to this general pattern. If unhelpful neighbours are present in any combination, even with just one other condition, then smoking rates are moderately high. Using chi square with a probability threshold of greater than 95% to find significant breaks in the range of smoking rates, three thresholds are evident as indicated by the plus signs in the table. These occur with the appearance of the first condition at the transition from a smoking rate of 10.3% to 19.0%, at the transition from 27.6% to 32.4% when unhelpful neighbours start to appear in the configurations, and at the transition from 46.5% to 56.8% when worklessness appears consistently in all configurations at and above this level of smoking. Configuration 6 is a slight anomaly as with all conditions present, including worklessness, it might be expected to have the highest smoking prevalence, but its rate is still very high.

Low income by itself is not concentrated among the high smoking rates, although it is more common among the configurations with the highest rates, probably because it is a consequence of worklessness. Low liveability does tend to be associated with higher rates of smoking, but only when in combination with unhelpful neighbours, no further education or worklessness. No further education appears to have little effect on increasing smoking rates because it spans a wide range of

Table 2.1: Qualitative Comparative Analysis of smoking configurations

No.	Workless	Unhelpful neigh- bours	No further education	Low live- ability	Low income	Smoking (%)	n
1	X	X	X		X	++++74.5	47
2	X		X		X	++++66.7	116
3	X		X	X	X	++++64.6	113
4	X			X	X	++++56.8	37
5		X	X	X	X	+++46.5	89
6	X	X	X	X	X	+++42.9	35
7			X	X		+++42.7	192
8			X	X	X	+++41.6	233
9		X	X		X	+++41.5	118
10		X	X	X		+++35.0	60
11		X		X	X	+++34.7	49
12		X	X			+++32.7	101
13		X			X	+++32.4	37
14				X		++27.6	105
15			X		X	++25.8	527
16			X			++23.9	331
17				X	X	++19.6	107
18					X	++19.0	126
19						+10.3	194

rates, and is only in the configurations with higher rates when combined with low liveability or unhelpful neighbours. Overall, the higher smoking rates appear to start with unhelpful neighbours, rise further with combinations of low liveability and no further education, and then reach their highest level among the workless configurations.

An implication of this analysis is that improving incomes and job prospects among disadvantaged communities may have a much greater impact than smoking cessation services. Measures to discourage smoking such as bans in workplaces and enclosed public spaces are important but may not impact on the inequalities gap if there are still opportunities to smoke in other contexts (Pickett et al, 2002).

Despite a sustained period of relatively low unemployment in the UK, worklessness remains a problem associated with long-term dependency on out-of-work social security benefits in areas of the country where demand for labour is not so strong and wages are relatively low. The transition from employment into worklessness is recognised as a risk factor for mental health problems but not for smoking, with which poor mental health is strongly associated (Thomas et al, 2005). Government programmes are now focusing on supporting people back into employment in these areas, and this may be an opportunity to offer support with giving up smoking at a time when smokers may be predisposed to giving up. Neighbourhood housing improvements may offer a similar possibility.

Why, however, should this predisposition occur, especially as waged employment may not offer an income appreciably higher than some benefits? Marmot (2004) observes that being excluded from employment is one of the most extreme ways to deny a person status and opportunities to exercise autonomy and participate socially with other people. Low status, low control and little social participation are, Marmot argues from a wide range of evidence, likely causes of emotional distress. They may be sufficient to activate biological stress pathways and encourage people to find relief by smoking. Of course, not everyone smokes under such conditions: 47% of workless people in the Middlesbrough sample did not smoke and neither did 66% of the low-income respondents. But for many it is a way to manage stress. Giving up can be left to when times get better. If the smoker's health is affected by continuing stress as well as the effects of smoking, there may be little motivation to give up because poor health may mean there is even less reason to make investments for the future (Lawlor et al, 2003).

If worklessness is one of the most extreme conditions of low status, control and social engagement, then living on a low income, lack of neighbourliness and living in a neighbourhood with visible deficiencies and problems seem likely to be similarly distressing. Their association with smoking was less strong than worklessness, but these conditions affect more people and, as already noted, when in combination had an effect on smoking similar in magnitude to worklessness. People whose smoking is an adaptive response to anxiety, depression or boredom are likely to find this behaviour reinforced by the processes of socioeconomic sorting that produce spatial concentrations of deprivation where smoking is acceptable among peers and part of day-to-day social interaction (McKie et al, 2003). In these conditions of circular causality, cessation is unlikely unless a positive life change means that future health is not so heavily discounted in favour of relief from present-day problems. This point is reflected in the evidence of how new hope and fresh starts can be a pathway to remission from depression (Harris, 2001). However, relapse is always threatening given the vulnerability of people in weak labour and housing market positions to repeated job loss or further exposure to neighbourhood problems.

The Middlesbrough results support this explanation, with smoking rates increasing as stressors are added to the configurations produced by the fsQCA analysis. While noting the limitations of cross-sectional data, there is reason to see this as an example of emergence. People are open, dynamic systems and adapt in ways that reflect their environments and the 'press' it exercises. Table 2.1 might be regarded as a simulation of different system states (the configurations of people–environment systems) and their emergent outcomes (the levels of smoking). Although the data are a snapshot, this approach invites us to think about moving through the configurations as transitions of system state. Whether this holds in reality would need further research with longitudinal data. But it was the configuration of smoking and lung cancer that ruled out a competing explanation at the time (the 1950s) that it was the hundreds of tonnes of tarmac being laid down across Britain that was to blame for the rising incidence of the disease (www.timesonline.co.uk/article/0,,60-1707232,00.html). Smoking was almost always present in any configuration of attributes of lung cancer patients.

Selection is a possible cause of the patterns in the Middlesbrough data, but selection has not been found to be a significant explanation for health inequalities in other studies. One longitudinal study of change in smoking prevalence following neighbourhood improvements found a sharp reduction in smoking, supporting the idea that it is poor living conditions rather than a selective filtering of smokers into these conditions that is the main process at work (Blackman and Harvey,

2001). Residents' mental health may influence how they perceive the liveability of their neighbourhood, and people in poor mental health are more likely to be smokers, but no evidence for this perception effect was found in studies by Latkin and Curry (2003) and Sooman and Macintyre (1995). In general, neighbourhood perceptions have been shown to correspond with observable physical features (Cho et al, 2005).

Further survey evidence would help to clarify whether the relationships found in Middlesbrough hold in other areas. It would be useful to have longitudinal data for people who move from worklessness into employment or from poor to better neighbourhoods. It would be particularly interesting to test the above arguments by evaluating interventions based on them. It would be possible, for example, to undertake a longitudinal study of programmes to move people into employment or renew neighbourhoods, following up their smoking behaviour. Whether smoking cessation services work better in these circumstances could be tested by comparing outcomes for programme beneficiaries taking up smoking cessation services with those where no special cessation advice or support are provided. If there is evidence of an additional health gain from combining NR interventions with smoking cessation services, this is likely to be a more effective way of targeting these services than simply focusing them on deprived neighbourhoods, which may well add to the stigma already experienced by residents.

Phase spaces and transitions

Initial conditions in neighbourhoods can make a considerable difference to what happens to them when something important changes in their wider environment. Nevin et al's (2001) work illustrates this very clearly and there are other examples. The effect on health of energy-inefficient housing may be masked during periods of low fuel prices when heating a home properly is affordable. It may become marked, however, with a rise in fuel prices. But a well-insulated housing stock with efficient heating systems is likely to considerably dampen the fuel poverty effects of changes in the energy-cost parameter: the prices of gas and electricity. In complexity theory, these different housing environments represent different 'phase spaces', which define the range of possible states for a system.

The possible trajectories for a system are contained within its phase space and new possibilities arise if this phase space transforms. One of the most significant transformations in the phase space of advanced capitalist societies has been a transition from 'organised capitalism' to 'disorganised capitalism'. The latter has been marked by the emergence of more flexible systems of production and a greater fragmentation of economic and social interests (Lash and Urry, 1987). This disorganisation of capitalism has been a disruptive force for many neighbourhoods, extremely so in the case of the disappearance of occupational communities such as mining and shipbuilding communities in the old industrial areas of countries like the UK. Neighbourhoods have adapted and been reorganised in the more fragmented image of disorganised, post-industrial capitalism. At one end of this spectrum are neighbourhoods of exclusion and worklessness, where local drug markets and crime emerged as a response to the loss of other economic opportunities, and at the other the gentrified neighbourhoods of exclusion housing the affluent post-industrial workforce of a services economy.

In keeping with the consumer rather than producer orientation of disorganised capitalism, housing markets have come to have a strong organising influence on neighbourhoods in post-industrial societies. This has been driven by processes of social filtering. In England, population migration shows a pattern of spilling down the settlement hierarchy from the bigger urban areas, to the suburbs, to small towns and then to rural commuting areas (Bate et al, 2000). This is overlaid by a north to south regional shift. These movements display a marked social dimension: it is the more affluent who lead the moves down the settlement hierarchy and from north to south, leaving behind less affluent and more deprived households. As Byrne (1998) remarks, neighbourhoods are both unique places and members of sets; every neighbourhood is different but the spatial sorting and filtering of people by class and ethnicity creates neighbourhood types.

These neighbourhood types, states or outcomes are emergent properties of the way the attributes of neighbourhoods and residents configure together as a system. This happens in a wider context that can be represented as a phase space. The type or state of a neighbourhood can be described in terms of multivariate coordinates in its phase space. These trace key parameters such as employment rates, housing demand and supply, environmental quality, public spending and so on. They also define the range of values which these variables can have given the economic, social and ecological limits of the larger system described by the phase space. Thus, a phase space can be transformed by a fundamental structural change such as the transition from national economies to open economies associated with globalisation.

Systems can follow a path marked by successive positions in this multidimensional space, or they may come to occupy a restricted part of the phase space, known as an 'attractor'. By way of illustration, Table 2.2 adapts Moobela's (2005) story of the regeneration of the Hulme area of Manchester to show how a neighbourhood can move through phase space in this way. The table shows the locations in agricultural, industrial and post-industrial phase spaces that Hulme and its different residents have occupied. What is apparent is that Hulme has undergone dramatic *non-linear* changes over relatively short periods of time in between longer periods of stability. These changes were associated with massive disinvestments or investments of resources. The periods of stability have been marked by different states, with each state one of a number of possibilities defined by the phase space of each era, from agricultural, to industrial and then to post-industrial phase spaces. There are, however, also important roles for self-organisation and interaction in what has been happening to Hulme, which have located the area uniquely within these phase spaces.

A key web of interactions for Hulme in the 1970s–80s was between a new but dysfunctional built form, a single mass housing tenure, the residualisation of that tenure by government policies and prevailing social attitudes about home ownership, and tenant organisation, all leading to an unmanageable mix of factors. These eventually found resolution through a range of local stakeholders engaging with the opportunities presented by new regeneration programmes, and leading to the transformation of Hulme into a culturally diverse mixed-tenure area. This all required self-organisation to happen, and took Hulme in one of a number of possible directions presented by the possibilities of its post-industrial phase space. Hulme's location in this space is as a 'mixed community', culturally diverse and widely regarded as a vibrant locality. Equally, the social divisions of housing tenure have not gone away but have been remade at a more fine-grained spatial scale than in the past (Meen et al, 2005). Whether mixed-income areas are stable attractors in this post-industrial phase space has yet to be established. Meen et al (2005) consider that there is a possibility that these areas will eventually tip back one way or the other, to either deprived or gentrified neighbourhoods, given that there has been no reduction in inequality at a societal scale.

Table 2.2 Hulme's trajectory through phase spaces

Time	State	Description
Pre-1760s	Attractor: agricultural area	Predominantly farming.
1760s–1890s	Chaos effect as connectivity transforms Hulme and it shifts to a new industrial attractor, with rapid in-migration of population to tightly packed terraces and courts.	A phase transition occurs with the Industrial Revolution, the key parameter change for Hulme being the connectivity that follows completion of the Bridgewater Canal to Manchester.
1890s–1950s	Population declines as Hulme morphs into an industrial slum, intensified by 1930s' depression.	High population density and unsanitary conditions create an unhealthy area of rampant infectious diseases.
1960s	Transition to a mass social housing attractor.	Wholesale slum clearance transforms Hulme over a few years into high-rise deck-access blocks of flats, dispersing the resident population and replacing it with a new population of social housing tenants. Redevelopment coincides with a phase transition from industrial to post-industrial conditions.
1970s	Post-industrial slum.	Deindustrialisation residualises new working-class social housing areas such as Hulme, compounded by housing policies favouring owner-occupation. Structural and design problems with the flats create a new unhealthy area of damp, vermin infestation, accidents, crime and vandalism. Families are moved out and replaced with single people. Tenants organise to press for demolition.
mid-1980s	Tipping point reached as Hulme enters a chaotic state.	Hulme acknowledged as 'unmanageable' and the council engages with residents to replan and redevelop the area again.
mid-1980s to present day	Hulme moves out of chaos to a new post-industrial attractor.	Hulme redeveloped as a mixed-use, mixed-tenure 'urban village'.

Source: adapted from Moobela (2005)

Conclusion: social space, geographical space and neighbourhoods

Hulme's population changed in a number of ways during this history. There were interactions between Hulme as a geographical space that changed and Hulme as a place where residents' location in social space changed. As Hulme became an industrial slum its working class changed, and changed again when it was replaced as a social housing estate. Its rebirth as a 'mixed community', however, represents an attempt to decouple social space and geographical space. Living in Hulme should no longer mean that a resident's location in social space can be deduced from their location in geographical space. Is this a good thing?

Results from the Joseph Rowntree Foundation's Mixed Income Communities programme suggest that most households moving into 'mixed communities' are either neutral or prefer them to other areas (Holmes, 2006). However, positive features of their environmental quality and safety, and access to 'good' schools, seem to be at least as important as their social mix. In terms of the latter, it is residents for whom the alternative may be a deprived social housing estate that may have most to gain. Even then, it could be the better environment and services that are important rather than the social mix. As discussed in the next chapter, it seems to be the 'press' exerted by the neighbourhood, and its interaction with individual attributes, that are important for whether we adapt to this experience in ways that are good for our health or bad. This adaptation includes abandoning environments of excessive press if we can, leaving behind those without the resources to move out. These residents may adapt to neighbourhoods of increasingly concentrated deprivation by focusing on short-term needs and fulfilment, in the absence of any long-term opportunities that are perceived as realistic. The resulting segregation of geographical space becomes sharper than people's differences in social space would suggest. The adaptation to short-term needs and fulfilment becomes judged by some in wider society as indicative of a lack of aspiration, whether manifested in drugs, smoking, eating unhealthy food or leaving education early to become a parent.

Mixed communities may help to prevent excessive press and these positive feedbacks of decline. There is no reason why low-, middle- and upper-income households should not share the same residential space; no one seems to lose out and some may gain. But this is not an outcome likely to happen out of individual choice in very differentiated housing systems. Gatrell et al (2004) show that people's attributes cluster in both geographical space and social space. Using the technique of correspondence analysis with survey data drawn from localities in North West England, they found two distinct clusters in social space among their survey respondents. The first was a socially stable cluster of home owners and older people who were keen to 'stay put' and willing to engage with neighbours. The second was a more unstable cluster with a lack of sense of community, a wish to move, a lack of engagement with neighbours, and a younger population. Gatrell et al overlaid geographical location on this social space, with the result that deprived areas and wealthier areas broadly segregated into different attractors, although by no means perfectly. Some people living in the deprived areas were located at an attractor in social space more typically occupied by people living in affluent areas, and vice versa. Overall, they found a broad division in socio-geographical space between the deprived and affluent neighbourhoods, but there was more heterogeneity across the deprived neighbourhoods.

Chapter One argued that the *extent* of this socio-geographical division probably does not reflect individual preferences but nevertheless arises from lots of individual choices. Policy has a role in establishing limits to how divided society can become, based on democratic mandates for societal rather than individual objectives. The policy objective of the NR strategy in England is not one of mixed communities but to establish floors below which no neighbourhoods should fall whether or not they are 'mixed', with these defined as relative gaps referenced to national averages. Although deprived areas in Britain are three times more likely to be considered noisy, four times more likely to be considered shabby, and less likely than affluent areas to be described as friendly, safe, green and with good local services, there is no simple linear relationship between deprivation and these negative evaluations (Collinge et al, 2005). Concerns are certainly more widespread in deprived areas, but for none of these indicators do more than 20% of residents living in deprived areas register negative evaluations. These residents are likely to be living in the minority of deprived neighbourhoods where liveability is a particularly acute issue. These are neighbourhoods where it is 'physical capital' that is having as much or greater effect on residents' own perception of their quality of life and opportunities as income-related deprivation, but where deprivation is likely to become increasingly concentrated.

The problematic areas are those of concentrated worklessness with poor-quality and often unsafe environments and poor schools and other services. These are also the areas most likely not to attract the private investment necessary to be transformed into a 'mixed community'. The state of health of their populations is a good guide both to their disadvantaged position and the potential for improvement. Evidence about what works to improve health at a neighbourhood level points to what measures need to be taken to renew these neighbourhoods as 'safe, green and clean'. This is the essence of a 'decent neighbourhood', the standard which currently does not exist and which therefore, unlike the 'decent homes' standard, has no target. Like the decent homes standard, however, it would need the investment necessary to achieve it, and a frank assessment – in partnership with residents – about whether some neighbourhoods can achieve it. The concentration of exclusion from work and education in the worst neighbourhoods means that public services need to be provided at a much higher level than elsewhere until levels of worklessness in particular drop to much lower levels. 'Mixed communities' are one way to do this, through new development or redevelopment, but this is not a feasible option for all the areas targeted by the NR strategy. We return to the issue in Chapter Four.

The NR strategy recognises that neighbourhood systems are nested in larger systems, and that the former cannot be isolated from the latter. Interventions are needed that recognise deprived neighbourhoods as emergent from wider processes of economic change and housing obsolescence, but with unique combinations of attributes in each place. The strategy is more than lots of local strategies, however, because it is framed in a national performance assessment framework that measures gaps in key indicators between the worst places and national averages. Health inequalities are likely in all societies with more than small income and wealth differences, so the issue is one of tolerable differences. This means setting targets, but it also means knowing how to intervene in complex processes. This understanding of how locally implemented strategies can be causally connected to national floor targets is as yet poorly developed.

Understanding health as an outcome of complex causation implies a research agenda aimed at identifying the attributes that affect health among the combinations of attributes in which everyone is embedded. If, as Ragin's (2000) fuzzy-set social science suggests, this points to patterns of necessary and sufficient conditions for health problems to emerge, then there is the potential to match national and local interventions to these conditions, using local knowledge to combine them in ways that can achieve qualitative rather than incremental change in neighbourhoods. A key objective of the NR strategy is to achieve a co-evolution across a number of fronts, such as worklessness, education and health, that can move neighbourhood systems out of deprivation at faster rates than national conditions are improving. The expertise required to do this is essentially that of matching appropriate programmes of additional resources and incentives to local contexts, breaking the links between mutually reinforcing 'bads', and creating win–win linkages between programme 'goods'.

There is a growing recognition in policy discourses of the complexity of wicked issues, and the need for changes in local governance to create capacity to intervene in causal combinations, rather than through the traditional silos of public services delivery. There is a challenge here for researchers to match this capacity with useful theory and evidence appropriate to this new governance context.

THREE

Emergence and environment press

Feedbacks and interactions: going upstream

Qualitative change in a system can arise from internal agency, an external intervention or more typically a mixture of both. At any given time, however, environmental parameters present limits to what is possible in a given phase space. Within these limits a variety of outcomes are possible, with local agency making a difference. The limits can also change with a phase transition. Take the example of a social housing estate in England. This housing tenure is nationally regulated in ways that create a defined space of possibilities, with limits defined by access to the tenure depending on housing need. Within these limits the range of possibilities for the local system state depend on the amount of local demand for social housing, the demographic composition of this demand, and the local response. These conditions can mean that a social housing estate is a settled, stable and popular place to live or an unstable and unpopular neighbourhood. In England tenants have the right to buy their rented properties and, as already discussed, many regeneration initiatives aim to diversify the tenure of social housing estates with more privately owned housing. At a certain point this extension of owner-occupation may change the parameters governing the state of the area and a *phase transition* to another state may occur; one in which new parameters such as mortgage interest rates take the place of previous parameters such as rent and subsidy policies. One consequence of such a change is that the neighbourhood may become more settled, with less turnover, but social housing opportunities will have been reduced.

Interactions between the agents in a system and with their environment have the potential to produce non-linear change or transitions to different *qualitative* states. This is what is meant by emergence: the outputs of a system are not proportional to the inputs – as with linear change – but are new states arising from causal combinations creating a qualitative change. Relations between agents and with their environment are therefore important in understanding the emergent potential of a system – the positions in the phase space it *could* occupy – especially how feedbacks have either a stabilising or transformative effect. Negative feedback maintains a stable state during which there is little or only incremental change in response to an input. Positive feedback produces a scale of change out of proportion to the input due to the multiplicative effect of interactions, potentially moving the system to another state. This is the 'tipping point' phenomenon (Gladwell, 2000).

Recognition of the transformative capacity of feedback distinguishes complexity theory from earlier system theories in the social sciences, notably the conservative functionalism of Talcott Parsons (1971). Positive feedback was evident in the case of Hulme's rapid expansion following completion of the Bridgewater Canal discussed in the previous chapter. Interactions with positive feedback can produce strong emergence such as gentrification, residential segregation, local crime economies or states of community health. These outcomes then become contexts for further interactions, which may either 'lock' the system into a relatively stable attractor with negative feedback or fuel a continuing process of change.

System responses to perturbations are feedbacks, and an intervention in a system is a type of perturbation. People, as agents, interact with the attributes of their environment, and an intervention aims to change one or more of these attributes to establish reasons or resources that can engender change. The attributes that appear to drive neighbourhood decline, for example, are crime, concentrated deprivation, successive waves of deprived incomers and poor environmental quality, but the extent to which these have causal power depends on wider processes of economic change and urban decentralisation (Nevin et al, 2001; Ecotec Research and Consulting Ltd, 2005; Green et al, 2005; Meen et al, 2005). The importance of these different drivers also varies from area to area depending on the neighbourhood's initial condition. It is when they act to reinforce each other in a process of positive feedback that a trajectory of decline can be travelled along very quickly, moving the neighbourhood through a phase transition to a different state that is difficult to reverse (Prime Minister's Strategy Unit, 2005).

Understanding the causal power of attributes, such as the level at which significant change occurs and whether attributes act on their own or in combinations, can point to where interventions may have success, how much input is needed, and how contextual features will work with or against the intervention. Thus, Meen et al (2005) argue that the best prospects for successful neighbourhood renewal interventions are in those areas that are not so deeply deprived that the available resources will not be able to get them to their 'take-off' points, when people with jobs and qualifications and private development will move in. In areas of extreme deprivation, where unemployment is compounded by high rates of long-term illness and lack of qualifications, the distance that needs to be travelled demands a considerable investment of public resources to get to a take-off point. These, however, tend to be very small areas within larger areas where the take-off point is more achievable.

A very deprived small area takes on more of the character of a closed system; literally a closed system if it reaches the point of abandonment and a static, maladaptive equilibrium. Intervention then has to move upstream to a control parameter if the area is to be moved from a position of long-term high dependency on public resources and poor outcomes for its residents. In the most depressed areas this means demolition and redevelopment. There is an analogy here with the concept of upstream and downstream interventions in public health, where upstream primary interventions change control parameters and reduce or remove the causes of outcomes downstream. Secondary interventions are more downstream and minimise the impact of these outcomes but are likely to have just incremental effects. Control parameters are upstream: they have the potential to engender changes in qualitative state.

Lifestyle interventions in public health are often regarded as upstream, such as tackling obesity with diet and exercise interventions, but they are a long way from being control parameters. Lifestyle interventions are generally time and labour intensive, using approaches such as behavioural therapies, incentives and support with attending sessions, but mostly have modest results (Jain, 2006). Moving up a level we can see that obesity has the same socioeconomic distribution as CVD, for which it is an important risk factor. At population level, sharp rises with decreasing occupational status are evident. Occupational status, and its association with material and psychological rewards, seems likely to be an order parameter for CVD (Brunner, 1996). Leyland (2005), however, argues from his analysis of Scottish data that it is area deprivation rather than individual occupational class that is associated with socioeconomic gradients in CVD conditions. This suggests that a more complex set of parameters may be behind the patterning of CVD, operating in causal combination.

Order parameters are powerful forces but are more likely to operate in causal combinations in a complex world than independently. This means that whether change in a parameter, and how much change, has an empirical or actual effect depends on how it combines with other attributes. This is also true of a system's collective variables, which may combine to engender emergence. Gatrell (2005) considers Buchanan's (2002) analysis of a syphilis outbreak in Baltimore, California. This epidemic broke out as a result of a combination of increased use of crack cocaine in the community, a cutback in medical services in deprived areas, and the dispersal caused by redevelopment in poor neighbourhoods of the city. Individually, none of these changes was dramatic, but in interaction they triggered a tipping point. Until this point, one infection was probably triggering just less than one other infection; after it, the disease was spreading in epidemic proportions. While it is easier to explain this phenomenon than to have predicted it, this explanation points to the importance of understanding how people adapt or *maladapt* to change in the environment. Preventative action upstream focuses on establishing the conditions for healthy adaptive behaviours. How we evaluate our futures seems to be central to this.

Adaptation and maladaptation: the importance of a future

Complex systems adapt through feedback by deploying resources to achieve outcomes, not least survival but also well-being and happiness. People are complex systems and if resources are limited their adaptive behaviours are far more likely to prioritise the short term because the long term is too uncertain. When resources are more available there is less need to prioritise short-term needs and greater incentive to invest in a more certain future to which it is possible to look forward. As Collinge et al (2005, p 10) comment, 'If people feel reasonably safe in their area and positive about their local environment, they will go on to focus on other things such as maintaining the positive aspects of what they already have'. This means, however, that in circumstances of resource scarcity, coping with immediate threats and meeting short-term goals is prioritised over making stage-setting moves that invest in the future (Chisholm and Burbank, 2001).

People adapt to adverse conditions but this can be in ways that are health damaging, such as smoking or drinking. The environment also adapts to people, such as local shops in poor areas offering few healthy food choices because most people cannot afford them. But there are still usually some choices being made, such as between buying cigarettes or apples, or having a baby at 16 rather than staying on at college.

Lack of resources is a major part of the picture but so are the reasons people have for what they do. If the living environment presents risk and uncertainty then the response may be to trade off long-term benefits to health against coping in the short term. The short-term offers benefits in the here and now, while the future is unpredictable.

Chisholm and Burbank (2001) draw on complexity theory to understand health-related behaviours in terms of our capacity to use internal models for evaluating future actions and selecting those that are most likely to be advantageous. They distinguish between people living in disadvantaged circumstances with limited resources and people living in advantaged circumstances with more resources. The latter group are likely to have a model of a worthwhile future, when they will be in good health, and therefore they select stage-setting moves that invest in this future.

Investing in the future is always to some extent devalued because it is always to some degree uncertain, so investing resources in stage-setting moves is more likely when the future is perceived as less of a risky prospect. Chisholm and Burbank (2001, p 207) comment: 'When an organism's future is uncertain, its most pressing adaptive problem has always been making sure that it *has* a future' (original emphasis). They develop this rather narrowly, however, in discussing teenage conceptions using the evolutionary concept of fitness and its translation into reproductive success. Their argument is that when current resources are very limited the rational behaviour is to produce offspring at an early age or high rate, investing minimally in each one given the probability that some will survive: '... when people lack the material or social capital to limit risk and uncertainty or to make a difference in their children's reproductive value, their optimal reproductive strategy will often be to maximise current reproduction – even at the cost of ill health, despair and shortened lives' (p 208).

This is clearly rather insulting to teenage mothers, who often respond to their new status by investing time in education and improving their job prospects. Above all, it ignores the way humans have to a great extent transcended biological evolution to embark on a journey of cultural evolution. Both types of evolution have a surprising amount in common, but not because of the zero-sum game between short-term and long-term investments that Chisholm and Burbank suggest. Evolution instead seems to reveal a dynamic that selects for non-zero-sum or win-win games engendered by the mutual benefits that flow from working together, such as divisions of labour, and which drive complex adaptive systems towards higher levels of complexity (Wright, 2000).

However, the Chisholm and Burbank hypothesis appears to have empirical support in that it is young women in the world's poorest countries that generally have high rates of reproduction, despite generally worse nutrition and health. Their hypothesis seems less convincing in developed countries, where the majority of teenagers in disadvantaged areas do not become mothers, but they suggest that attachment theory offers an explanation here. Most young people enjoy responsive and caring social relations beginning in infancy that are likely to translate into secure, positive and helpful 'internal working models'. These in turn shape romantic, sexual and parenting relationships in adulthood. Some, however, do not and experience abuse and neglect. This is not to deny the role of adverse environments, but to identify why some young people are more vulnerable than others to environmental stress (there is a possible link too between the activation of stress hormones and the early onset of puberty).

Warm and responsive caring has an anti-stress effect. It is not surprising, therefore, that evidence points to certain groups of young people being especially vulnerable to becoming teenage parents. They include young people in or leaving care, homeless young people, those excluded from school, truants and underachievers, children of teenage mothers, and young people involved in crime. Abuse by adults is a common theme in their bibliographies (Swann et al, 2003). There is a strong relationship with deprivation, but this is likely to reflect both the effects of deprivation on some young people – and their possibly abusing parents – and the spatial sorting into deprived areas of young people coping with these vulnerabilities. If you are experiencing exclusion and low self-esteem then this will be compounded by living somewhere few others would live in out of choice. Seeking motherhood as a defining identity, and the doors to both state and family support this is likely to open, becomes a rational alternative (Graham and McDermott, 2006).

Further evidence on this issue appears in an article by Cohen et al (2000) on sexual health. They calculated rates of gonorrhoea cases for housing blocks in New Orleans and found a strong relationship with a 'broken windows' index measuring housing quality, abandoned cars, graffiti, litter, and public school deterioration. The 'broken windows' phenomenon is known to have a number of effects, including on health, that are independent of measures such as neighbourhood poverty. Cohen et al found that their index explained more of the variation in gonorrhoea rates than a poverty index measuring income, unemployment and low education. A high broken windows index on its own was a sufficient condition for high gonorrhoea rates, whether or not this was combined with a high poverty index. As with other cross-sectional studies of this nature, the causal relations involved can only be speculated upon, but it seems that depressing and disadvantaged neighbourhoods may create contexts for high-risk behaviours, and that these may be less likely to be checked by other residents, who respond to the area's problems with pessimism and by keeping themselves to themselves.

Ganz (2000) makes a similar argument in proposing that people – and indeed public policy – are likely to focus on ameliorating the most immediate risks posed by their environment, and it is only when the most immediate risks are dealt with that more distant risks, which are now more immediate, get attention. Efforts aimed at reducing threats to personal safety or property in neighbourhoods where personal safety or property is perceived to be at risk could encourage people to reduce or stop smoking because they are less likely to face these more immediate dangers. They can, therefore, enjoy the benefits of better future health because more pressing and troubling conditions have been dealt with.

Health as an emergent property and tracer of underlying social problems

The person–environment system is not reducible to its parts. Yet intervention often assumes this. For example, a first step for community health projects is often to compile a 'community profile' by auditing lots of separate things. This could include data on the prevalence of serious illnesses and risk factors such as physical activity, smoking, stress, birth weight and teenage conceptions; socioeconomic data such as benefit claims, ethnicity and languages spoken, levels of employment and education; and data about the quality of housing and public spaces, opportunities for leisure and play activities, crime rates and local transport. This is then compared with the services provided for the neighbourhood and who is accessing them, with the aim of identifying gaps in provision or the way services are provided, such as opening hours.

None of this can be profiled as if the neighbourhood is a closed system. Important results can be achieved from these exercises, but they tend to be reductionist snapshots in time, producing 'shopping lists' of needs that even if met may not achieve any long-term change. A complexity approach instead aims to identify the parameters that are affecting the state of a neighbourhood and their causal combinations, and to intervene more upstream.

The liveability of neighbourhoods is one such parameter: the visible environmental quality of residential surroundings or its 'physical capital'. This is a perspective often reflected in residents' own assessments of what needs to be done. A recent MORI study of liveability, for example, reports that:

> [W]hen talking spontaneously about these issues [the local environment, safety and community] people link them all together in intricate ways, with virtuous and vicious cycles very evident to residents. For example, it is common for residents to feel that problems with crime need to be resolved before the environment can be improved in a sustainable way, but at the same time feel that characteristics of the local environment encourage crime. And both of these elements in turn help encourage or destroy feelings of community, which itself is seen as vital to improving local areas. (Collinge et al, 2005, p 20)

The report continues: 'What other people think of their area is important to people, particularly as it implies something about the residents themselves' (p 22). The importance of interactions and feedbacks between problems such as crime and the environment, or between residents as trusting neighbours or suspicious strangers, comes over clearly from these findings. So does the relational nature of how we see ourselves and our circumstances.

In a neighbourhood, all parts of the local situation enter into the situation as active participants. Neither a resident nor their residential environment exists independently of their encounter with each other (Ittelson, 1973). Greenery, for example, may be perceived quite differently in an affluent area compared to a poor area, as uplifting and good for property values in the former but threatening and a hiding place for muggers in the latter. Whether a neighbourhood is perceived as a good or bad place to live will depend on how normal we see our current neighbourhood compared with other worse or better places. The effect of these comparisons will in turn depend on the discrepancy we perceive between where we live and where we think we should live.

People who live where they want to live are likely to behave differently to people who live where they think they should not have to live. Explicit or implicit rules and norms of behaviour arise adaptively as collective variables. In a high-crime neighbourhood many residents may adopt a rule of not going out after dark, and in doing so continue to reproduce a perceived if not actual state of unsafe streets at night (a negative feedback; a positive feedback would be residents using the streets after dark to reclaim them, with the possibility of a transition to a safer state). In a safe, affluent neighbourhood, a norm or rule of behaviour may be to intervene in minor incivilities that affect the 'tone' of the neighbourhood; a type of behaviour described by the term *collective efficacy*, which itself is an emergent property. The previous chapter considered smoking as an emergent property: people who are workless and live in stressful neighbourhood conditions smoke 'as a rule'. In the absence of these conditions people do not smoke 'as a rule'. The behaviour has a routine nature but also variability: not everyone who is poor smokes, and not everyone who smokes is poor. But there is enough emergence to create a collective variable with causal implications, notably the strong relationship between deprivation and premature mortality at the macro-scale caused by smoking-related illnesses.

While the prevalence of smoking in a neighbourhood is an apparently simple product of individuals who smoke compared with those who do not – and is therefore apparently reducible to individuals – the fact that such a high level of smoking occurs in certain conditions is not amenable to a reductionist analysis. Furthermore, reducing health-related behaviours to single dimensions such as smoking or unhealthy diets fails to recognise both the clustering in the same individuals of unhealthy behaviours due to underlying causal factors such as deprivation and stress, and the feedbacks between these behaviours. For example, a smoker who successfully stops smoking may find relief from a stressful environment by eating more as their appetite increases with not smoking. As they put on weight, their risk of obesity-associated health problems increases (Adams and White, 2005).

People–environment interactions therefore produce 'population health', an emergent property beyond reduction to individual causation, and often a tracer of underlying social problems. In Lefebvre's (2000) terms, however, population health tends to be constructed in 'representational space'. This is the conceived space of 'officialdom' used to collect data, organise services or allocate resources; it is also the space of epidemiology. Lefebvre's alternative concept of 'lived space' is produced by people in their everyday lives and is the realm of community health. This is the health that emerges from spatial practices and local habitus. Community health is reducible neither to the individual nor collective because it is relational. Even '... what is assigned as an individual level variable at one time point could equally be conceptualised as a characteristic of past environments in which those individuals grew up' (Sundquist et al, 2004, p 75). Not only are the effects of various aspects of the environment *embodied* over time, but environments are embodiments of human practices.

Every person who becomes very ill or dies is a story of individual suffering and loss, but there is also a 'big picture' of illness and premature death that traces the *condition of a society*. Marmot (2004, p 255) comments: 'If health suffers it tells us that human needs are not being met. Health may be a condition, but inequalities in health are telling us about more general social inequalities in the crucial influences on health'. These influences, and their health effects, are structured by class, gender, ethnicity, neighbourhood and other 'group properties' that we can use to help explain observed patterns in society (Archer, 1995). Despite the current English health policy agenda being summed up by the recent White Paper title, *Choosing Health*, with its emphasis on 'making healthier choices easier', many people feel that their health is affected by factors beyond their individual control (DH, 2004a). This is more likely to be perceived as the case among low-income, socially excluded or BME people who will be hard to reach with conventional public health campaigns. A straightforward example of this is choosing a healthy lifestyle. Using modest assumptions, Morris et al (2000) calculated the cost of a healthy lifestyle for a single male aged 18-30 and found that it exceeded the UK's minimum wage by £12 a week (at 1999 prices). In 2005, this gap was probably around £20 a week (Deeming, 2005).

Income, however, is only part of the picture and needs to be considered in relation to the wider environment and the incomes of others. The epidemiological transition, which occurred around the middle of the 20th century, was an environmental change and not just a response to a growth in incomes. The transition marked the point when the developed world reached a standard of living and public health that meant that infections were less likely to start and spread. Life expectancy has continued to rise as the quality of living has risen and as working and living environments have improved in ways that make them less hazardous, from health and safety regulations to central heating in homes and better fridges and freezers. It is these *qualitative improvements* rather than just rising income that appear to be behind the epidemiological transition, explaining why improvements in life expectancy level off with further increases in income over time in countries that have passed through the transition (Wilkinson, 1996).

It was improvements in working and living environments that engendered the epidemiological transition, but these environments are again raising concerns about new epidemics in developed countries.

These include asthma and allergies, obesity, diabetes, heart disease, depression and other mental illnesses. The epidemiological transition means that we are in a new phase space, but emergence is still apparent in a range of new public health threats that reflect types of maladaptation. Individual lifestyle often appears as the most immediate cause, but these new problems show patterns and trends that suggest a structuring by environmental conditions.

Alcohol-related morbidity in the UK is an example. Alcohol is increasingly contributing to mental and behavioural disorders, liver disease, poisoning, accidents and circulatory diseases. It is also a driver underlying crime, and a factor in 50% of street crime, 33% of burglaries, 30% of sexual offences and a third of domestic violence offences (NRU, 2005a). The rate of alcohol-related deaths in England and Wales doubled over little more than 20 years between 1980 and 2003, from 6 to 11.6 per 100,000 population (ONS, 2005b). Figure 3.1 shows a strong relationship between alcohol-related deaths and local area deprivation. There is also a regional dimension. With the exception of Brighton, the highest death rates occur in local authority areas in North West England. The rate for the North West, 15.1 deaths per 100,000 population, is almost double that for the East of England, with 7.7 deaths per 100,000 population. This difference is reflected in hospital admissions. Table 3.1 contrasts emergency admissions for alcohol-related illnesses in the Strategic Health Authority (SHA) area of Cheshire and Merseyside in North West England with those in the Norfolk, Suffolk and Cambridgeshire SHA in the East of England. The rate of emergency admissions for mental and behavioural disorders due to the use of alcohol is more than three times higher in Cheshire and Merseyside. Across the North West, alcohol consumption is driving a widening life expectancy gap between deprived and non-deprived areas, cancelling out the narrowing of this gap that has been achieved by a falling death rate due to smoking-related causes (Wood et al, 2006).

Alcohol-related deaths are expected to increase in the coming years and may cancel out much of the health gain achieved from falling rates of circulatory diseases and cancers, but the cause is not clear. There is a strong association with area deprivation, a link which a US study by Hill and Angel (2005) suggests is partly explained by heavy drinking palliating anxiety and depression arising from living in disordered neighbourhoods. However, alcohol consumption is greater among people with higher incomes (ONS, 2005b). People on higher incomes who report high levels of stress also tend to drink more, but this does not seem to be reflected in outcomes for their physical health

Figure 3.1: Alcohol-related deaths and area deprivation, English local authorities

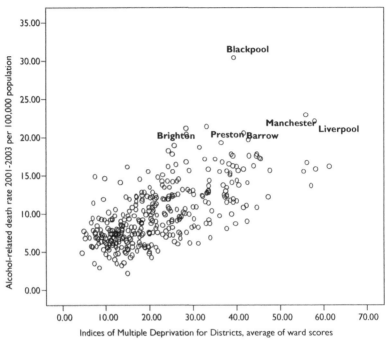

Source: National Statistics

Table 3.1: Alcohol-related emergency admission episodes per 100,000 population, 2003-04

SHA of treatment	Mental and behavioural disorders due to use of alcohol	Alcoholic liver disease	Toxic effect of alcohol
Norfolk, Suffolk and Cambridgeshire Strategic HA	36.7	16.76	2.93
Cheshire and Merseyside Strategic HA	124.6	30.79	3.06

Source: Parliamentary Written Answer, 20 July 2005

(Heslop et al, 2001). There seem, in other words, to be two epidemiologies of deprivation- and affluence-related causation, but with different consequences depending on vulnerability arising from socioeconomic position and its effect on material disadvantage.

Evidence from Middlesbrough suggests that falling unemployment in a town that is still highly deprived may increase heavy drinking as young men acquire more disposable income, possibly combined with competitive alcohol promotion campaigns by bars and nightclubs (Anderson, 2005). Certainly there is a gap in current public health targets, which do not address alcohol consumption, and a need for more research on the cause of the UK's emerging problem, especially when in some other countries alcohol-related deaths are declining.

Environment press, ageing and dementia

Hill and Angel's (2005) argument that neighbourhood disorder encourages heavy drinking is an example of Lawton's (1980, 1982, 1989) concept of environment press. This is an idea that has considerable general relevance to this book's arguments, from offering explanations for the epidemiologies of smoking and alcohol consumption, to exploring the environmental exclusion of people with dementia. Dementia may seem an unusual topic in this context, but it ranks with other emergent conditions on this side of the epidemiological transition as one of the dominant epidemics of the 21st century.

Lawton developed the idea of environment press in his work on physical environments and ageing, but it has general application (Scheidt and Windley, 2003). Lawton argued that psychological well-being is greatly influenced by the ability to maintain a sense of control over our immediate living environment. He saw this as an interaction between an individual's ability to cope with the challenges posed by an environment and its demands or 'press'. Press has positive value, providing benefits of environmental stimulation and challenge that are good for psychological well-being. So, applying this to the alcohol example in the previous section, it may be that too much environment press, without the ability to cope with it adaptively, increases the risk of maladaptive strategies like heavy drinking, explaining the association with deprivation. Too little environment press, perhaps because affluence can insulate people from risk and surprise, engenders the same heightened risk of excessive drinking, but this time inversely related to deprivation. Smoking may not follow the same pattern of two epidemiologies because nicotine is an anti-depressant for when times are difficult, and non-smoking an established norm in affluent circles.

This is a speculative application of Lawton's concept but we are on surer ground considering his ideas in relation to older people. His theory of ageing and disability recognises the association of these conditions with declining levels of competence in adapting to environment press. There is a greater likelihood of unfavourable outcomes because of this loss of adaptability, and press starts to have a negative effect unless the environment is adapted. Lawton argued, however, that people's need to explore is as strong as the need for security. This does not disappear as a result of loss of competence, suggesting how oppressive it may be to confine older people if they have impairments to a 'safe' indoors. Even indoors, stairs are treated as a hazard for older people rather than as a way of continuing to promote physical activity, with their safety an issue of design rather than presence or absence (Shipp and Branch, 1999). For Lawton, living environments should provide a range of environmental options, which he believed to be enriching and of value to mental and physical health. Indeed, this chimes with the evidence on how job strain can arise from either excessive demands or too little job latitude, but in interaction with individual characteristics and coping resources (Marchand et al, 2005). 'Liveable' environments may be free of health-damaging stressors but they are not bland and without 'soul' (Collinge et al, 2005).

Lawton gives surprisingly little attention to the outdoor environment, being mainly concerned with housing. There are in fact very few studies of the effects of neighbourhood conditions on older people, despite the likelihood that they spend more time at home, rely more on local services and have greater emotional attachment to their home than people in younger age groups. There is evidence that environmental satisfaction and neighbourhood sociability are important influences of older people's sense of well-being and their functional independence (Glass and Balfour, 2003). Results from the Alameda County Study in the US suggest that neighbourhood press may influence functional loss at older ages (Balfour and Kaplan, 2002). Excessive noise, inadequate lighting and heavy traffic were particularly significant risk factors for subsequent deterioration of ability to undertake physical tasks such as climbing stairs.

It is being discouraged from going outdoors that is likely to be behind this loss of independence. Poor-quality or unsafe neighbourhood environments are particularly likely to influence the participation of older people in outdoor activities. Yet going outdoors is important not just for independence in carrying out activities such as shopping, or for the pleasure of taking a walk, but also to maintain health through physical exercise and contact with nature and other people.

Physical or cognitive impairment can mean that the outdoors presents too many barriers compared to a safer and more familiar indoors, effectively disabling people because of poor design, planning or neighbourhood management, and even confining them to their home. For people with a condition such as Alzheimer's disease and other less common dementias that lead to disorientation and difficulty with comprehension, the navigability and legibility of environments becomes a challenge. A person with dementia is as much a complex adaptive system as anyone else in the sense that, despite a loss of adaptability, adaptation occurs – but often as an avoidance of disabling environments. Like smoking as an adaptation to an adverse environment, avoiding disabling environments is a maladaptive response. This is not just because of the loss of quality of life that follows from environmental exclusion, but also because the lack of outdoor activity and stimulation is likely to *contribute* to functional decline.

Although disability rights activists have pressed home the message that impairment is not 'abnormal' but part of the range of human variation that should be accommodated by inclusive design and planning practice, cognitive impairment has been neglected. This is despite there being about 750,000 cases of Alzheimer's disease in the UK, with this projected to increase to 870,000 by 2010 and 1.8 million by 2050 as the UK ages (www.alzheimers.org.uk). This scale of impairment among the population is not dissimilar to the number of wheelchair users in the UK, estimated at around 750,000 (Harrison et al, 2004). But the level of knowledge and awareness about how dementia becomes disabling because of environmental barriers, and how non-disablist assumptions in planning and design can discriminate against people with dementia, is far behind that of wheelchair use.

The 2005 Disability Discrimination Act (DDA) amended the 1995 DDA to require all public authorities to promote disability equality, including that of cognitive impairment. For planning and highways functions, the issue is invariably conceptualised as one of standards of access for people with mobility and sensory impairments, with no consideration of the needs of people with dementia. Yet the emphasis of UK health and social care policy is to maintain people with longer-term needs in the community, including providing care closer to home (DH, 2006b). This is not only the option wanted by most older people, but when people with dementia move from their own home to a residential or nursing care home, their risks of depression and an earlier death are heightened (Day et al, 2000). Institutional care can have a disabling effect that, while perhaps unavoidable with severe dementia because of the extent of risk, needs to be delayed for as long as feasible.

There is also a marked contrast between the lack of evidence, regulations and guidance about outdoor environments for people with dementia and the numerous design guides that have appeared since the early 1980s offering planning, architectural and interior design recommendations about *indoor* care settings for people with dementia, such as day care centres and nursing homes (Day et al, 2000). Much of this guidance is based on research and, while this enables some hypotheses to be formulated about what might also be the case outdoors, there has so far been only one study that has looked at this issue directly (Mitchell et al, 2003).

Dementia brings with it progressively declining abilities to plan a route, remember or try different options, recall earlier mistakes, remember or use real or mental maps, and use spatial information and signs (Blackman et al, 2003). Support with understanding what to do in a particular context, such as finding somewhere to rest or posting a letter, and with finding the way around places, has the potential to re-able people with dementia despite their cognitive impairment. Maintaining a sense of control over the immediate physical environment is important for everyone's psychological well-being but becomes a sharper issue with age-related functional decline, both physical and cognitive.

Lawton (1989) differentiated between three functions of the environment: *maintenance*, or the constancy and predictability of the environment; *stimulation*, or the presence of novelty in the environment; and *support*, or the extent to which the environment compensates for reduced or lost competencies. We still know very little about how environments function in these ways for people with dementia. Maintenance is the function that is most understood because of a need for environments that support familiarity and communicate meanings clearly (Mitchell et al, 2003). The redesign of public telephone boxes, for example, to facilitate their use by wheelchair users may discriminate against people with dementia if the new design removes the traditional design features that communicate the function of a public telephone box to someone with dementia.

Lawton's particular contribution is his emphasis on stimulating environments and on not removing all challenge and novelty from 'adapted' environments. Evidence for this is well documented in Zeisel et al's (2003) review of the effects of physical environments on the behaviour of people with dementia in long-term care homes. Walking paths with features of interest along the way have been found to decrease exit seeking from the home and improve the mood of residents. Gardens have also been found to reduce elopement attempts and aggression, improve sleep, and engage family members with residents. Common spaces that are homely have been found to reduce social withdrawal. An ambience with meaningful and understandable sounds, sights and activities has been found to reduce agitation. Privacy has been linked with reduced aggression and agitation and better sleep. Overall, a residential rather than institutional character to the home is associated with reduced social withdrawal, greater independence and improved sleep, as well as more family visits.

There is a danger, however, that these adapted environments are separate spaces in which people with dementia are confined not out of their own choice but because professionals and family members are concerned that they should be safe and comfortable. Lawton's work emphasises both assistive adaptations to compensate for impairment and opportunities to interact with an environment that offers some challenge, interest and stimulation. Two implications follow from this. First, people with dementia may be able to relearn how to function in a range of surroundings if they have the opportunity and support to do so. Second, it may be possible to extend what has been learned about environmental adaptations and cues to support indoor living to adapting the outdoor environment of neighbourhoods, shopping centres, parks and other public spaces. Otherwise, the world and the challenge, interest and stimulation that it offers are likely to shrink for people with dementia, living in residential and nursing homes or, as most continue to do, their own homes in the community, cut off from the outdoors.

In Chapter Two, I suggested that the QCA output could be regarded as a simulation of what might happen to smoking rates if certain smoking-inducing attributes could be removed from the social and physical environment. Computers are powerful tools for simulations, providing the means to explore scenarios and model emergence from interacting attributes. The facility to model and display actual physical environments extends this to being able to explore the interaction of a person with a simulated urban environment, investigating issues such as legibility and wayfinding. The technology can put the user 'in control' and simulate an experience of *place* (Portugali, 2006).

It is only in recent years that research into the needs of people with dementia has treated them as active participants, able to speak for themselves rather than have carers and professionals speak for them. However, the accounts of people with dementia will often not be reliable for a range of reasons, from wanting to appear as fully competent as possible to memory difficulties. While dementia presents particular issues in these respects, these are by no means unique to people with dementia, and one solution is also not unique: to observe what people actually do rather than what they say.

People with dementia are already being involved in exploring design ideas and testing prototypes of aids such as tap and gas cooker monitors (Orpwood et al, 2004). Testing the wider environment is more difficult, however, because it is not so easy to test prototypes. Mitchell et al (2003) at Oxford Brookes University have carried out the world's first study to involve people with dementia in talking about how the planning and design of outdoor environments either helps or hinders them by undertaking accompanied walks outdoors. They make a number of planning and design recommendations based on this feedback but have not been able to test actual adaptations. In the real world it is rarely possible to redesign a road crossing just to test whether it works better for someone with dementia. But what about using virtual worlds?

I am currently leading a research team that is using the University of Teesside's computer facilities for generating semi-immersive virtual environments (VEs) to test actual planning and design changes with people with dementia. A computer-generated VE can be relatively easily adapted by changing the computer model to incorporate design changes such as better signage or different colours, enabling a participant to repeat their walk in the adapted setting. The resulting person–environment interaction can be observed and the performance of various tasks compared pre- and post-adaptations.

Computer-generated VEs have been used to create dynamic three-dimensional images for the assessment and rehabilitation of people with functional and cognitive impairments (Rizzo et al, 2002). A key feature of these environments is that a user can interact directly by using an interface device such as a joystick, moving through the VE as if really there, an experience called 'presence'. The study reported here, which is ongoing at the time of writing, is using a virtual reality model of Middlesbrough town centre that runs on a personal computer platform and projects onto a large curved screen in a small auditorium, together with ambient street sounds. The town centre was accurately recreated using a 3D modelling and animation software package, and the model transferred to a visualisation package for display in the auditorium. Participants sit close to the screen and control their navigation through the VE using a joystick. The model is very detailed, with pavements, kerbs, signs, road markings, a range of street furniture, pedestrians and moving traffic.

Participants are older men and women diagnosed with mild to moderate Alzheimer's disease or vascular dementia and with no significant physical or sensory impairment. In the first stage of the project they undertake two walks: one through the virtual town centre and one through the real town centre to test for any differences in response. This check on the validity of participants' virtual experiences has shown that the model is a reasonable simulation of the real town centre except for awareness of oncoming traffic when crossing roads, which is impaired by the restricted peripheral vision in the VE.

As participants walk through the town centre they are engaged in a structured conversational interview that takes them through a series of tasks that are scored for how successfully they are undertaken. The tasks include finding a specific street, crossing a road to find somewhere to sit down, finding a post office, finding a taxi, navigating through a shopping precinct to find a bus station, finding a specific bus stop, and finding a public toilet. The performance of each task is assessed in terms of the legibility of environmental elements, such as recognition of seating and its function, the destination challenges and how much prompting is needed to achieve them, participants' perceptions of the ambience and attractiveness of different places, and the awareness they show of safety considerations.

One of the most consistent findings at this stage in the research is the importance of clear signage designating what things are, such as 'bus station', 'telephone' and 'toilet', and the prominent listing of bus numbers at bus stops. Sequences of signs are also important – on the way to a public toilet for example – giving reassurance to participants that they are still heading the right way. Elements deliberately added to the VE as landmarks did not help with wayfinding. Participants found it difficult to associate a landmark with a destination, although some recognised things that were familiar to them individually, taking reassurance from this that they were in the right place. Most participants found no difficulty with navigating a variety of road crossings and were very cautious of traffic, although a potential danger was confusion about shared surfaces where vehicle ways were not clearly distinguished from pedestrian pathways by different surfaces and curbs. Traffic was widely disliked and the most popular space was a pedestrianised shopping precinct with seating and clean, spacious areas. Aspects of urban design that might be expected from the indoor research to pose problems, such as coloured paving patterns and modern street furniture designs, were not problematic outdoors except for some problems recognising seats and telephone boxes for the most cognitively impaired participants.

Our findings do not support encouraging older people with dementia to walk outdoors on their own in unfamiliar environments. They were mostly accompanied by carers. But it is still important that a person with dementia can interact with an environment so that it provides stimulus rather than strain, and a more fulfilling experience for both the carer and the person with dementia.

Dementia and complexity

Ageing is often characterised as a loss of adaptability. One of the discoveries from looking at how complex systems adapt is the role of fractal structure, which is a repeating pattern at multiple scales (Lipsitz and Goldberger, 1992). Adaptive structures have many fractal dimensions, giving them a 'bushy' look. Processes can also have a fractal character, displaying many aperiodic fluctuations within an overall pattern, and these processes appear to be able to adapt to change in their environment more successfully than regular, mechanical processes. Ageing is associated with a decline in the complexity of the brain and a fall in its fractal dimensionality, due either to an impairment of functional components or a disruption in how these components couple together. This appears to cause a loss in the dynamic range of brain processes. The effects of this loss of complexity in the person with dementia's brain are a diminished ability to remember what happened in the recent past, to engage in goal-directed behaviour into the future, and impaired capacity to absorb, store, recall and use new information. This can be summarised as a reduction in the capacity to deploy *schemata* as mental schemes or behavioural structures for carrying out tasks such as walking to a destination or crossing a road.

People with dementia, however, still use schemata, at least in the mild to moderate stages. This implies a need for assistive adaptations that provide simple and focused components or elements in the environment. These should help with specific tasks by removing the environmental load that does not contribute to schema acquisition and maximising that which contributes directly to constructing cognitive schemata (Van Gerven et al, 2000). People with dementia also have difficulty combining tasks and are easily distracted, again implying environmental adaptations that do not require combined tasks and limit distractions by supporting schemata acquisition without too much cognitive load. In Alzheimer's disease, the most common type of dementia, the impairment of episodic memory – memory of personally experienced events – but the retention of semantic memory of vocabulary and general facts about the world, also point to adaptations such as clear word signs and generic rather than novel designs for street furniture or entrances, exits and crossings.

Adapting an environment to the capacities of a person with dementia aims to compensate for this loss of complexity, especially by simplifying environmental signals and reducing environmental stressors. However, in line with Lawton's argument, this should not be to such an extent that the remaining complexity of the person with dementia's brain is not exercised by environment press. Environmental adaptations should encourage cognitive activity and in doing so may help slow the progression of dementia and achieve a degree of 'rementing' in response to stimulus (Kitwood, 1997; Rizzo et al, 2002). Environmental adaptations therefore need to get the balance right between environments for people with dementia that are not excluding because of overdemanding press, and environments that still offer a level of press that is stimulating for a brain that has lost complexity.

There is also a strong public health argument for getting this balance right so that the outdoors is inviting for people with dementia. As well as the physical health benefits of even low-intensity exercise such as walking, there is evidence that the more that older people walk and take exercise the less their risk of dementia (Abbott et al, 2004; Scherder et al, 2005; Larson et al, 2006). There are several possible explanations for this, such as the effects of walking on cognitive activity and links with cardiovascular health. The former explanation is supported by a study by Weuve et al (2004), which found that older women who are more physically active, including walking, had better cognitive function across general cognition, memory, fluency and attention and, in effect, aged more slowly. Women with cognitive impairment who walked more also experienced less cognitive decline. As well as having a preventative effect, walking may slow the progression of dementia.

This perspective is very different from a medical model that reduces dementia to a diseased brain. Lawton considered ageing and age-related conditions in a transactional perspective in which neither a person nor an environment has any independent existence because both exist in a people–environment whole of mutually causal feedbacks. But he returned to an interactional perspective because of the difficulty of operationalising this transactional idea empirically (Wahl and Weisman, 2003). An interactional perspective treats behaviour as an outcome of the characteristics of the person, their environment and an interaction between the two. It is possible to both operationalise these influences as variables for quantitative analysis and model the causal mechanisms. Thus, 'although person and environment form a unified system where what is inside is philosophically inseparable from what is outside, for heuristic purposes, it is necessary to speak of, and attempt to measure, them separately' (Lawton, 1998, p 1).

As I have already argued, Ragin's QCA is an attempt to deal with this problem. In QCA, cases are not regarded as preconstituted. They are contingent configurations of attributes with diverse possible outcomes. QCA is a method and not a theory, however, and it is complexity theory that can help with a theoretical framework because the contingent configuration of attributes that constitutes a 'case' is an open, dynamic and adaptive system. If we work with this concept, then the theory leads down particular paths of explanation about where to look, what to look for, and what sense to make of what is seen. Complexity is essentially about interaction and its consequences; it is not cases and attributes in themselves that are important, but the relations among attributes and the patterning of outcomes for cases. Someone with Alzheimer's disease will experience a range of disabling symptoms but the outcome depends on how these configure with their environment and the care they receive. Kitwood (1997) emphasised particularly that those 'behavioural symptoms' of dementia labelled as 'aimless wandering' or 'aggression' are more likely to occur in certain configurations where there is distress or discomfort caused by their surroundings or other people's behaviour. I have argued earlier that smoking can be considered in similar terms. These are behaviours that should not be considered, let alone 'treated', outside the configurations that are the generative processes.

Conclusion: the buoying environment

Environments that marginalise people and reinforce disempowerment and disability are environments that deny 'personhood'. Personhood, according to Kitwood (1997, p 8), is 'a standing or status bestowed upon one human being, by others, in the context of relationship and social being. It implies recognition, respect and trust'. Space is socially produced, so that spaces that cause stress, disable their users or are under-stimulating are *acts* done by some to others. The personhood of people who have to live or work in these spaces has been denied by others who will often live in spaces that signify recognition and respect of *their* personhood. People are more likely to fall ill and die early in these circumstances.

Travelling through London earlier today I was struck when passing a high-rise social housing estate by children's bicycles crammed into the small balconies of the flats. Clearly an adaptation to nowhere else being safe to store these bikes, it was also a small but significant marker of what has to be coped with when the environment is not adapted to the way of life of people living there. Lawton's work on environment press has a lot to offer in understanding this people–environment 'fit'. Lawton argued that there needs to be a balance between people's competence – from children's ability to ride bikes to a person with dementia's ability to wayfind – and the 'press' of the environment: the stimulation and support it offers as a place to ride a bike or get out to the local shops. Environments can be harmful because they are too demanding or because they demand too little.

The theory is, as Glass and Balfour (2003) remark, of the 'use it or lose it' school. However, these authors argue that Lawton overemphasises press or challenge, and that this needs to be balanced by considering attributes of the environment that are supportive and which 'buoy' individual competencies. Figure 3.2 draws upon Glass and Balfour's model, incorporating their concept of environmental buoying as at the positive pole of the press scale. Smoking status and physical activity are included as examples of outcomes. The attributes are system parameters, including liveability, neighbourliness, design and local services. Their effects are modelled as press or buoying. The former includes a range of possible stressors from crime to noise, physical barriers, and the in/accessibility and quality of services. The latter includes the effects on well-being and control of liveability and neighbourliness, environmental prosthesis, or how design supports competence and facilitates adaptation, and support from other residents and local services. An interaction is included between these effects and personal competencies.

These competencies include attributes such as impairment, coping resources in the form of income, education or family support, and personal coping styles, with health as an emergent outcome or system state. There is, of course, far more going on than is depicted at the level of Figure 3.2. Hereditary factors are part of the picture, other settings such as the workplace are involved, and living standards, the distribution of income and wealth, and the effects of climate change or other natural hazards need to be considered for any truly holistic model of health. What Figure 3.2 seeks to capture is how pathways to health outcomes operate at a neighbourhood level: 'It is through these pathways that the balance of press, buoy, and competence *get into the body* to affect functioning and health' (Glass and Balfour, 2003, p 322; original emphasis). The next chapter turns to consider the first part of the diagram, the attributes of neighbourhoods that affect our health.

Figure 3.2: Causal model of the neighbourhood system

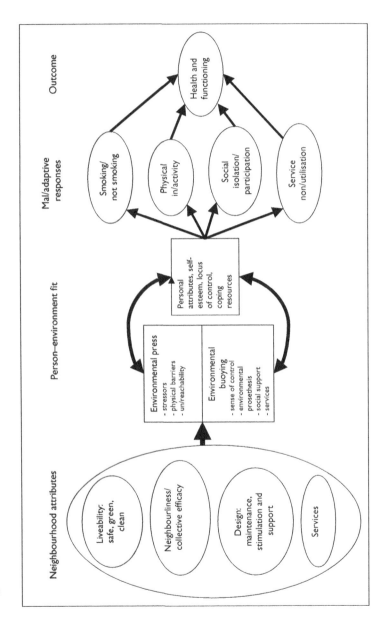

FOUR

The neighbourhood effect

It is often argued that communities of propinquity, neighbourhood communities, have declined as people's work and consumption patterns have become wider and more fragmented (Gilleard and Higgs, 2005). This transition has been described in various ways, such as from Fordism to post-Fordism, from 'organised' to 'disorganised' capitalism, or from modernity to late modernity or post-modernity (Lash and Urry, 1987). In the UK, this new phase space is post-industrial. But although the occupational basis for a neighbourhood identity such as that of a pit village or shipyard community may have largely disappeared, neighbourhoods still often have a material basis in consumption terms. The collective consumption of shared space also takes on a special meaning when it is centred on the home, a place of emotional, financial and labour investment, and where a sense of personal identity and value may be very influenced by how much the neighbourhood is in demand as a place to live. The neighbourhoods of consumer society may be different from the neighbourhoods of industrial society, and part of people's wider and more numerous networks in a more complex society, but they remain meaningful systems, and systems that have effects.

Neighbourhood effect studies

Community studies based largely on qualitative methods have a long history of exploring the distinctiveness of 'places' and testing general theories of social change by 'grounding' them in specific places (Crow, 2002). In recent years, there has been an expansion of quantitative investigations of whether variations in outcomes such as educational attainment, voting, health status, children's behaviour and domestic violence can to some extent be explained by variation between small-scale geographical contexts once differences between individuals are controlled for statistically. This statistical modelling separates 'individual' from 'neighbourhood' effects, and in general suggests a much larger effect on health of individual-level variation than neighbourhood-level variation (see Kawachi and Berkman, 2003, for a comprehensive review). Even so, spatial strategies such as ABIs may be able to achieve an appreciable global health gain if they can achieve an improvement in health across large numbers of people.

The evidence about only a small compositional neighbourhood effect is not conclusive. A study by Leyland (2005), for example, suggests that it is area deprivation rather than individual occupational class that is associated with socioeconomic gradients in CVD conditions. He argues that it may be the aggregated characteristics of neighbours rather than individual characteristics that are important, such as living in areas where a lot of people smoke, and smoke more heavily.

Propper et al's (2005) study of neighbourhood compositional effects on mental health is one of the studies that points to a small neighbourhood effect. They constructed bespoke neighbourhoods of about 500-800 people around individual survey respondents in the British Household Panel Survey, using population census data to profile the neighbourhoods. Five dimensions of neighbourhood conditions were examined, using composite measures in multi-level models and exploring non-linear and interaction effects. Using self-reported symptoms as assessed by the General Health Questionnaire (GHQ), they found that variance at the neighbourhood level accounted for less than 1% of the between-individual variation in both levels of, and changes in, the prevalence of common mental health problems. Women and people from BME groups or who had a low level of education appeared to be more affected than average by characteristics of the neighbourhood, but these effects were still small. By contrast, individual and household characteristics of SES, ethnicity, gender and housing tenure were significant influences on mental health, although these factors did not predict future mental health.

Neighbourhood compositional effects, therefore, seem to vary by health outcome as well as across individuals. There are difficult methodological issues with identifying what effects neighbourhoods really have. These include obtaining data about both individuals and their neighbourhoods, and defining the neighbourhood when this is limited by the geographical units for which data are available. Incomplete adjustment for individual SES is another problem (Reijneveld, 2001). The neighbourhood itself may also influence individual SES, such as individuals being advantageously positioned in relation to employment or educational opportunities. Neighbourhood effects may not be apparent across all socioeconomic levels, and particularly adverse or particularly advantaged neighbourhood conditions may be the issue, with threshold rather than continuous effects.

Pearl and Pickett (2001) suggest that neighbourhood effects may not be so apparent in countries with less polarised neighbourhoods compared to countries with a high degree of neighbourhood polarisation. However, a study from Sweden, a reasonably egalitarian country, has demonstrated marked neighbourhood effects on the incidence of admission to hospital for CHD (Sundquist et al, 2004). This large-scale multi-level study included all Swedish men and women aged 40-64 years in 8,547 neighbourhoods of around 1,000-2,000 people. Individual characteristics included in the statistical models were age, gender and income, and neighbourhood characteristics were measured by an area-based deprivation index used to allocate primary health care resources. The risk of developing CHD was found to be 87% higher for women and 42% higher for men in the most deprived neighbourhoods compared to the most affluent. This was after accounting for individual income, which also had a strong significant effect, and both neighbourhood deprivation and individual income displayed gradients in terms of CHD outcomes.

The role of social capital

Socioeconomic level as a parameter begs the question of what it is about aggregate SES, beyond the individual, that may have effects on health. Among the possible explanations are socio-cultural features of the neighbourhood, the area's reputation and contextual conditions likely to be associated with average socioeconomic level, such as the quality of the physical environment including air and water, healthy home, work and play environments, and levels and quality of local public and private services (Macintyre and Ellaway, 2003). Stafford et al (2001) found that, among their sample of London civil servants, neighbourhood problems such as noise, unsafe streets or fewer local facilities, along with defective housing, explained some of the relationship between area deprivation and health. They did not find that increasing area deprivation was associated with more restricted social networks, but comment that they could not measure the quality of social interaction.

A number of studies have considered how the quality of social networks, participation, cohesion and support affects health. These are different dimensions of 'social capital', a concept that describes social or family ties and participation in community activities that support a sense of belonging, reciprocity and trust in others. Putnam (2000) argues, deploying a wide range of evidence, that social capital has a strong influence on health status and that measures of social capital correlate with morbidity and premature mortality independently of the effects of material deprivation. The evidence, however, is not consistent. Mohan et al (2005) found no relationship between mortality and synthetic estimates of social capital they were able to calculate for electoral wards in England. They conclude that material deprivation remains the most likely explanation for geographical variations in health. Despite this, there is a significant number of studies that suggest a link, particularly with circulatory diseases and children's behaviour. The evidence for mental health is more mixed.

Two pathways for how social capital might affect health are through buffering stress or influencing either health-related behaviours or actual health states directly (Kawachi and Berkman, 2003; Cohen et al, 2006). Social support may be part of the explanation, and there is an extensive literature about the positive effects on health of social support from family members, friends or neighbours (see Callaghan and Morrissey, 1993, for a review). These effects can be both direct and indirect, such as the influence of having supportive friends on encouraging physical activity (Parks et al, 2003). Neighbourhoods may also be important contexts in influencing whether the effects of social support operate, since Elliott (2000) found that social support only buffers individuals from stress in high SES neighbourhoods. But there is also something distinctive about social capital compared to social support, despite obvious overlaps, and this is related to notions of social cohesion and trust between people, shared norms and values, informal social control, and engagement in community and civic life, all of which are potentially neighbourhood attributes.

Neighbourhoods, however, are only one framing of the networks that may supply social capital. Many people are less dependent on neighbours for social support and their networks less locally based than in the past. Lindström et al (2006) found that adults' psychosocial conditions *at work*, the job demands and job latitude, are strongly associated with their degree of social participation, including activities beyond work itself such as sport, church or large family gatherings. Poortinga (2006) argues that the health benefits of social capital do not exist 'out there' so that, for example, someone in poorer health could move to a neighbourhood high in social capital and see their health improve. Although trust and social participation may be individual rather than collective attributes, there is always likely to be interaction between these levels. Poortinga finds that in countries where there is a high overall level of trust, those individuals with higher levels of trust or participation in social activities are more likely than low trust/participation individuals to report good or very good health.

But in countries with a low overall level of trust, they are less likely to do so.

A distinction is sometimes made between cognitive social capital and structural social capital, with different measures used in empirical studies. The former concerns perceptions such as trust and sense of belonging, while the latter is about engagement and participation. De Silva et al's (2005) systematic review of studies of social capital and mental illness published up to 2003 uses this distinction, and considers separately studies that measure social capital at an individual level and studies that do so at a geographical level. For the former, they conclude that there is strong evidence that common mental disorders decline as levels of cognitive social capital increase, although the evidence is less strong for children. The issue with this finding, however, is the causal direction: mentally ill people are more likely than others to appraise things negatively and withdraw socially, so there is no reason to favour an explanation that it is weak social capital which is a risk factor for mental ill-health. There is also evidence of an inverse relationship between structural social capital and mental illness at an individual level, except for one study reporting a positive association.

At a geographical level, De Silva et al (2005) found mixed results but overall no clear evidence for an inverse relationship between the level of social capital and mental illness. Two US longitudinal studies pointed in opposite directions: one finding that high levels of social capital were associated with a decreased risk of suicide among discharged veterans, and the other that high levels of social capital were associated with lower levels of recovery from alcohol dependence among homeless mentally ill patients. Social capital may work in different and interactive ways to produce these different outcomes. De Silva et al (2005) suggest that higher social capital neighbourhoods may take a supportive attitude to deserving cases such as veterans while being much less tolerant of homeless mentally ill people.

A review of the literature on social cohesion and social capital by Stafford et al (2005) identifies eight dimensions: family ties, friendship ties, participation in local organised groups, integration into the wider community, trust, attachment to neighbourhood, tolerance and being able to rely on others for practical help. In a study of neighbourhoods defined as postcode sectors of around 5,000 people in England and Scotland, they found that these measures of social cohesion were closely correlated with crime and with the local political environment as measured by voter turnout and left-wing voting. These could be distinguished statistically from local amenities and more physical aspects of the residential environment. Worse scores for both types of factor were associated with poorer self-reported general health. The effects were found to be stronger for women than for men.

Overall, trust appears to be the aspect of social capital most important to at least mental health, but it is difficult to separate this effect from concomitant feelings of being unsafe in what can be comparatively violent neighbourhoods, certainly in the US (Kling et al, 2005).

Drukker et al (2003) report a multi-level analysis of relationships between the health and behaviour of 11- to 12-year-old children living in 36 'ecologically meaningful' neighbourhoods in Maastricht and neighbourhood levels of social control. Children's mental health and behavioural problems were significantly worse in neighbourhoods with low levels of informal social control, which also tended to be areas of residential instability. These were generally deprived areas where, according to the authors, 'informal social control agents ... may show a tendency not to correct aggressive and acting out behaviour in children because of feelings that children must be able to defend themselves through such behaviour' (p 836). However, some neighbourhoods with high informal social control were also highly deprived, while some with low social control were not deprived areas.

It is possible that low levels of informal social control by some adults in disadvantaged neighbourhoods follow from their own feelings of powerlessness and alienation that can accompany concentrated deprivation, with this then feeding through to a lack of responsiveness from local services (Wilson, 1996). This not only means that the local environment deteriorates but also increases the risk of antisocial behaviour and crime among local young people, some getting their sense of connection and community from gangs rather than failing parents, schools or workplaces. McCulloch (2006) found that in Britain the statistical effect on children's behavioural problems of living in a deprived urban ward was as great as for family-level factors. He suggests that lack of safety may be behind this relationship, with children exposed to violence and having their own activities restricted by a fear of violence.

There is evidence that some types of social capital can be *bad* for health. Stafford et al (2003) found that high family ties were associated with greater odds of worse health among women, although not among men. Stead et al (2001) suggest that the neighbourliness and attachment to local area they found among people living in disadvantaged areas of Glasgow encouraged high levels of smoking. These communities had 'strongly pro-smoking norms' and smoking expressed identification and belonging in its collective aspects of sharing, lending and borrowing cigarettes. Parkes and Kearns (2006) found that respondents who reported friendly people or good neighbours were more likely to report their health as 'not good'. Community involvement, however, was linked to better health.

Other evidence that social capital may be bad for health is a study by Wen et al (2005) of mortality among hospitalised older Chicago residents. They found that local social network density was detrimental to survival following serious illness and suggest this may be due to associations between higher levels of social network density, more crime and violence in the neighbourhood, and lower SES. These effects of close social networks chime with Putnam's concept of 'bonding social capital', which describes networks of people with much in common and a strong orientation inwards to family and immediate neighbourhood (Putnam and Feldstein, 2003). The inward–looking nature of bonding social capital contrasts with 'bridging social capital', which describes ties between different types of people across a greater social distance. Other work suggests that a combination of strong bonding social capital and weak bridging social capital has a negative effect on health independent of other influences such as SES (Almedom, 2005).

Putnam and Feldstein (2003) regard bonding social capital as a common outcome of 'birds of a feather flocking together', but identify a role for community development to facilitate building bridging capital where there are not the economic resources for this to emerge. While health policies that address social capital, mainly in mental health promotion, do not tend to differentiate between types of social capital such as bonding and bridging capital, they do tend to emphasise participation in social life. The UK Social Exclusion Unit's report on mental health, for example, advocates improving access to opportunities for volunteering, sport, art and leisure activities, roles in the community and participation in social networks (SEU, 2004).

Wen et al (2003) warn, however, that economic investment cannot be ignored in favour of social capital explanations and strategies. Jobs, decent benefits and services are needed, not just 'community development'. Low income will restrict opportunities for autonomy and social participation that are important for good health, regardless of where a person lives, and is associated with a greater fear of crime independently of whether the neighbourhood is deprived or not (Pantazis, 2000). But geographical concentrations of low incomes do create additional vulnerabilities such as no shops selling good food, children with little money getting involved in antisocial behaviour or crime, and a stigmatising of the area making it difficult to obtain employment or to recruit teachers for the local school.

Many deprived areas may only experience these problems occasionally or not at all, but they are more likely to than non-deprived areas, and the effects may serve to compound the damage to health caused by lack of autonomy and social engagement by reinforcing these problems at an environmental level. Nevertheless, community development can be an important foundation for economic development, building on existing networks of social ties and trust relationships, and achieving a critical mass of people committed to the same objective. Putnam and Feldstein (2003) present a collection of case studies that demonstrate this process unfolding in some US localities. Equally, community development has the potential to build bridges beyond neighbourhoods of exclusion, to link them into the wider economy and with other groups working on similar issues.

As well as community development, interventions could include using design and planning to promote social interaction. High residential densities, mixed land uses and gridded street patterns are possible means of maximising social contact between people as well as promoting physical exercise (Jackson, 2003). There is some particularly interesting evidence about the role of greenery in this respect, which is reviewed later, but overall the evidence base to support any specific social capital interventions to tackle poor health is not very good (De Silva et al, 2005).

This paucity of evidence is not stopping design and planning ideas being put into practice. In England, the level of demand for new housing in the wider London region is leading to the zoning of large greenfield areas for new residential development. The Communities Plan, as already noted, is a strategic policy framework for planning large-scale greenfield development in the South of England while renewing old urban areas in the North. This divided picture regionally tends, however, to be more mixed at the local level and the proposed new settlement of 'Harlow North' in the East of England is a good example (Ropemaker Properties Limited, 2005). Twenty-five thousand new homes are planned as an extension of Harlow, a relatively depressed early post-war new town in need of regeneration. The proposed new settlement is based on 13 connected neighbourhoods of relatively high-density housing and mixed uses, with people living within six minutes' walk of neighbourhood services. Among the many concepts that inform the master plan are 'living streets':

> All the streets are designed to be useful routes, lined with front doors and overlooked by windows, rather than blind cul-de-sacs lined with back fences and gardens. Such streets

are safe and lively. They discourage crime and break up the
monotony of traffic. And they are great places to live, cycle
and walk. (Ropemaker Properties Limited, 2005, p 21)

The evidence for such claims is ambiguous. Jackson (2003) cites a US
case of neo-traditional on-street housing where residents reversed the
design concept of overlooking the street by planting shrubbery to
block views from the street and protect privacy. It is by no means clear
that people prefer gridded street patterns to loops and culs-de-sac
despite some evidence that the former encourage sociability. In addition,
while the heavy sustainability emphasis of the Harlow North proposals
is likely to reduce its ecological footprint significantly, it is a strategy
designed to win planning permission for large-scale greenfield
development. Harlow North is also being designed as a socially mixed
settlement with 30% of new homes available at rents and prices
affordable to those on low and middle incomes but integrated with
other properties. This also, however, makes commercial sense given
that planning permission is more likely because of the emphasis on
affordable housing as planning gain in national housing and planning
policy. Indeed, these social and environmental goals may be better
achieved by infilling and redeveloping the existing Harlow urban area,
possibly a less attractive marketing prospect.

Concentrated affluence and mixed communities

Harlow North is being designed to avoid either concentrated affluence
or concentrated deprivation, and it is significant that achieving health
gain is part of the concept for the development. It is also noteworthy
that the relative deprivation that has emerged in the original new
town has stigmatised the area and led to population loss. In Chapter
Two the role of concentrated deprivation as a driver of out-migration
was considered, but just as we also saw that key parameters governing
neighbourhood abandonment appear to be more associated with
increased affluence than increased deprivation, it also appears to be
the case that the compositional effect on health of SES at
neighbourhood level may have more to do with concentrated affluence
than concentrated deprivation.

Unravelling the effects of concentrated deprivation on the one hand
and concentrated affluence on the other is not straightforward. It is
much easier to identify programmes that have aimed at redistributing
the poor than redistributing the well off. One of the former, the US's
Moving to Opportunity programme, has been extensively evaluated

using a randomised controlled trial research design (Kling et al, 2005). Poor residents in high-deprivation public housing schemes in five US cities were offered entry to a lottery for rental vouchers to move home. These were almost all female-headed one-parent households of black or Hispanic ethnicity. Applicants were randomly assigned to one of three groups: a voucher valid only in low-deprivation neighbourhoods, a geographically unrestricted voucher, and no voucher (the control group). Follow-ups after four to seven years found that among adults who were able to move to low-poverty neighbourhoods there were no effects for adults' employment, earnings or benefit dependency.

The experiment did not seem to be working as a means of achieving better economic outcomes, but it *was* working as a means of improving health outcomes. Adults reported significantly less psychological distress than those who remained in high-poverty neighbourhoods. The effect was comparable to some of the most effective clinical and pharmacological mental health interventions. There was also a large effect on obesity, possibly linked to the reduced psychological distress and an increase in exercise and nutrition. There was no significant effect on adult physical health. Among young people (aged 15-20), girls were found to benefit significantly from moving to less distressed neighbourhoods. Mental health, education and the likelihood of risky behaviour all improved, together with a small effect on physical health. Among boys, however, outcomes were *worse* in the experimental groups. Health, school achievement and risky behaviour deteriorated. The reason is unclear, with a possible explanation being that boys who moved often found their new environment more stressful.

Are these effects of leaving behind concentrated deprivation or living among relative affluence? The presence of affluent households in a neighbourhood has been linked to raising the overall health of a local community separately from any effect of deprivation. A study from Chicago shows that, for a given neighbourhood, a 10% increase in the proportion of households with annual family incomes of $50,000 and over was associated with a 10% increase in the odds of residents reporting better self-rated health (Wen et al, 2003). The study found that, at the neighbourhood level, affluence is more powerful than either deprivation or income inequality in influencing health, suggesting that *some affluence in all neighbourhoods* is an important contributor to community health. Other studies have found that the cognitive and emotional well-being of children and adolescents are correlated with the proportion of higher-income families in a neighbourhood, and have no relationship with the proportion of low-income families (Curtis, L. et al, 2004).

The causal mechanisms behind these relationships are currently poorly understood. The presence of more affluent households appears to be linked to a higher likelihood of resident intervention in neighbourhood problems, contributing to a neighbourhood's *collective efficacy*, which is a type of social capital. An influential idea in the US is that neighbourhoods of concentrated deprivation lack the collective efficacy of middle-income neighbourhoods necessary to keep problems such as antisocial behaviour, drugs misuse, littering and dumping under control. Thus, collective efficacy describes the capacity of a local population to self-regulate and control deviant behaviours and visible signs of disorder, with residents feeling empowered to intervene in trouble without risk of retaliation, and to demand and expect responses from public services. Poor people, it is argued, are less willing or able to intervene or put pressure on agencies to respond effectively out of a sense of powerlessness and pessimism. Concentrated disadvantage may in fact create a neighbourhood effect by reducing individuals' levels of perceived efficacy, but the evidence on this is mixed (Boardman et al, 2001).

Positive effects of affluence have been found for neighbourhood safety, cohesiveness and the overall helpfulness of neighbours, and problems such as rubbish and drugs. Wen et al (2003) found that two indexes of community social resources and physical environment largely explained the association between self-rated health and concentrated affluence at the level of 343 'neighbourhood clusters' in Chicago, after adjusting for social, demographic and behavioural factors at the individual level. The index of community resources measured collective efficacy and social network/reciprocated exchange. The collective efficacy scale combined responses to such statements as 'people around here are willing to help their neighbours', 'people in this neighbourhood can be trusted' and 'you can count on adults in this neighbourhood to watch out that children are safe and don't get into trouble'. Social network/reciprocated exchange was measured by combining answers to questions about friends in the neighbourhood, get-togethers and exchanging favours among people. The physical environment scale combined answers to questions about litter, graffiti and vacant buildings. Wen et al argue that neighbourhood economic context might work through social resources to influence health. In a later study, results are presented that suggest that collective efficacy may derive its protective effects on health primarily by reducing crime, violence and victimisation (Wen et al, 2005). This study was confined to a sample of older Medicare patients in Chicago, and points to neighbourhood safety as a key parameter influencing post-hospitalisation mortality.

A very important caveat from this study, and research on neighbourhood effects in general, is that individual low income is persistently detrimental to health, even when living in an affluent neighbourhood. Stafford et al's (2005) analysis of English and Scottish survey data found that the percentage of variation in self-rated health accounted for by between-neighbourhood differences was, for men, only 4%, compared to 96% within neighbourhoods. The between-neighbourhood variation for women was slightly higher at 6%. While this appears to make neighbourhoods relatively insignificant settings for health improvement, closing the gap in neighbourhood effects will benefit large numbers of people in ways that are likely to make a noticeable difference to their quality of life. Even at an individual level, analyses of risk factors leave most of the variation in health outcomes unexplained.

There is a parallel here with school improvement research. A recent analysis of test results for schools in England indicates that about 8% of the variation between schools in results is accounted for by a 'school effect', after taking account of a range of student and school contextual factors, such as prior achievement and income-related eligibility for free school meals (DfES, 2004). Yet this effect is the focus of major programmes to improve educational achievement, especially among students from disadvantaged backgrounds. The effect being targeted by school improvement interventions is relatively small but it accounts for a range in performance across schools equivalent to one and a half years of student progress.

Although individual and family characteristics such as income are still much more strongly associated with health outcomes than neighbourhood characteristics, unraveling these relationships is difficult and risks making false distinctions between people and places (Macintyre and Ellaway, 2003). No people–environment system is predictable. Neighbourhoods with low deprivation can lack cohesion and informal social control, just as neighbourhoods with high deprivation can have high levels of cohesion and social control. So although an absence of affluent households appears to increase the risk of neighbourhood problems, the effect is not inevitable (Drukker et al, 2003). However, in identifying attributes that increase the likelihood of better community health, this research does point to the possibility of significant health gains to be had from turning around problems of neighbourhood disorder, both physical and social. Achieving a better social balance, now very much on the UK's regeneration agenda, primarily by ensuring that at least some properties in a neighbourhood are attractive for 'middle-class' home buyers, seems likely to be beneficial. Indeed, 'mixed' or 'balanced' communities is now a common theme of British housing and planning policy, although by no means a new one.

Mixed communities, residential segregation and population mobility

The general trend in the UK has been one of increasing residential social segregation by social class and ethnicity, and this segregation is most marked at neighbourhood level. There are increasing examples of mixed income neighbourhoods with new development and regeneration incorporating this principle but they are a small proportion of the total housing stock. The trend towards greater segregation reflects rising income and wealth inequalities since the 1970s and their interaction with a spatial sorting of households by property markets into desirable and undesirable neighbourhoods, the effects of competition for 'good' schools, and the allocation of the poorest households to the 'worst' social housing estates or private landlord housing, where vacancies are most available (Babb et al, 2004; Berube, 2005).

The continuing expansion of owner-occupation as tenure of first choice in the UK, leaving social housing as a tenure of last resort, has created a general geography of ownership and non-ownership of housing wealth. In regions such as the North East of England, where large amounts of social housing were built to improve working-class housing conditions in the decades between and after the two world wars, housing policy now aims to reduce this tenure's share of the housing stock and increase owner-occupation (NEHB, 2005). While this reflects popular aspirations, there is a risk of home ownership expanding too far, with lower-income households becoming vulnerable to arrears at times of high interest rates, or having insufficient resources to keep their properties maintained – both with potential health consequences. There is also already some evidence in the North East of shortages of social housing, especially among younger households. Unfortunately there can be antisocial behaviour problems associated with these households, impacting on the already less popular estates where they tend to be housed, and worsening the liveability and sustainability of the area.

Expanding owner-occupation in social housing areas, either through redevelopment or sales to existing tenants, is one way of stabilising neighbourhoods that have become more unstable as social housing is increasingly occupied by more transient households. Deprived areas in general tend to have a more mobile population than other areas, presenting challenges for area-based social programmes. For example, in Sure Start areas more than one in ten residents moved into the area only in the previous year, while nearly 10% moved out (Barnes, J. et al, 2005). In some areas this turnover is much higher, at a quarter to a third of the population. Sure Start staff are continuously having to reach new families with young children while others move away. Regeneration can also promote selective population out-migration, particularly if residents who gain employment decide to move out to a better area. An evaluation of a training programme in Harlesden, West London, run as part of a City Challenge regeneration scheme, found that while people who moved out of the area had an unemployment rate of 9%, those who moved in had a rate of 21%, and those who stayed a rate of 15%. The effect was that unemployment was higher at the end of the programme than at the beginning, although not because the programme itself had been unsuccessful (Berube, 2005). Clearly these issues apply as much to area-based health improvement programmes.

Few studies have taken into account population mobility in investigating relationships between neighbourhood conditions and health. This is an issue given that a person's current health status may reflect circumstances connected with a previous neighbourhood of residence, such as unhealthy housing conditions in childhood. An independent effect of a deprived area in childhood on later adult health is reported by Curtis, S. et al (2004) in their analysis of data from the ONS Longitudinal Study for England and Wales. Monden et al's (forthcoming) analysis of survey data from Eindhoven in the Netherlands found that childhood socioeconomic environment and neighbourhood socioeconomic environment later in life were closely related. Despite being linked, they both independently predicted smoking and being overweight, controlling for individual socioeconomic characteristics. Similarly, Marsh et al (1999) found from their analysis of longitudinal data from the British National Child Development Study that both past and current poor housing conditions have independent effects on current adult health. Poor health among people living in non-deprived housing conditions was partly associated with housing deprivation earlier in life. Moreover, multiple housing deprivation – encompassing poor physical conditions, poor amenities, low satisfaction and past homelessness – was very hazardous to health, and the greater or more sustained this deprivation the greater the likelihood of ill-health. Overall, Marsh et al estimate that, among the National Child Development Study cohort, who were born in 1958, the impact of multiple housing deprivation was similar to that of smoking on health and greater than the effect of excessive alcohol consumption.

It is also likely that healthier people will tend to migrate to less deprived areas, while less healthy people will tend to gravitate towards more deprived areas, given the relationship between SES and health. In England and Wales, selective migration has been shown to have a marked effect on what appears to be the health of a place. Norman et al (2005) analysed data from the Office for National Statistics' England and Wales Longitudinal Study to investigate this issue by testing whether, over the 20-year period from 1971 to 1991, there had been any systematic spatial sorting of healthy and unhealthy people according to area deprivation. The health measures used were limiting long-term illness and mortality. They found that over this period there had been a substantial accumulation of healthy people in the most affluent electoral wards and a reduction in all other wards, while those who moved into the most deprived wards were significantly less healthy than people already living in these areas. They also found that people who lived in wards where the level of deprivation improved between 1971 and 1991 had significantly better health at the end of the period than people living in areas that remained at the same level of deprivation. In general, migration was found to increase inequalities in health between the most and least deprived wards, and to be a more important cause of change in an area's health status than change in the level of deprivation associated with residents who did not move area.

Residential social segregation in the UK has not reached the extremes apparent in the US. With the recent shifts in policy towards planning requirements for new developments to be mixed tenure, investment in improving social housing to the decent homes standard, the continuing promotion of the 'right to buy' for social housing tenants, and measures to target the lowest-achieving schools for improvement, there is a chance that the effects of these sorting processes can be modified. The HMR initiative in England has a strong focus on redeveloping low-demand, low-income housing areas as mixed-income neighbourhoods. However, it is difficult to attract home buyers to depressed localities and the best prospects for mixed developments are in areas of market strength (Holmes, 2006). Private developers of 'mixed communities' also favour grouping low-income rented housing separately from private housing for sale rather than fully integrating it. Planners also need to have regard to household types in these developments so that there are, for example, enough families in privately owned housing that send children to local schools. Schools need to be sufficiently socially mixed to avoid the stigma that can be acquired by only serving predominantly disadvantaged areas.

In the US, the federal HOPE VI programme has funded the demolition of rundown public housing schemes and their redevelopment as more mixed-income neighbourhoods. Overall, only about half of the original residents have been rehoused in the same neighbourhood and relocated residents receive assistance with moving to another estate or vouchers that subsidise them moving into private rented accommodation. A tracking study has found that, for most residents, their housing environment improved as a result of the programme, but a substantial proportion experienced continuing problems with drug trafficking and violent crime, and about half of those who moved into private renting using the vouchers found it difficult to pay the rent (Buron, 2004). Also, while the intention was to encourage rehoused residents to participate in new, more supportive social networks in mixed-income areas, relatively little interaction with new neighbours occurred.

If the theory that neighbourhoods lacking more affluent, empowered residents have deficits in collective efficacy is correct, there may nevertheless be other ways in which these deficits can be tackled than trying to change the social composition of a local area. One candidate is improving neighbourhood services so that they are more responsive and intervene when there are early signs of problems. This is the concept behind the expansion in England of Neighbourhood Management, Neighbourhood Wardens and Community Support Officers. There are likely to be almost 25,000 Community Support Officers within the next few years, supporting the local police with a high-visibility patrolling and enforcement role. Neighbourhood Wardens are employed by local authorities, social landlords and voluntary agencies, and have more of an environmental and mediation role than Community Support Officers. Both are very popular with local residents.

The underlying issue, therefore, is the liveability of the neighbourhood and the extent to which this either presses or buoys. Antisocial behaviour, violence, crime and environmental disorder are key aspects of liveability. Neighbourhoods with these problems are likely to affect many people's sense of control and self-esteem, especially if there is a dissonance between the environment they would like to experience beyond their front door and the environment they encounter.

Liveability and the green neighbourhood

An absence of significant hazards to health as assessed by the Housing, Health and Safety Rating System forms one component of the decent homes standard (Battersby et al, 2002). Considerable capital spending is currently being targeted on renewing the housing stock in England with the aim of all social rented housing meeting this standard by 2010. This is a significant step forward in protecting low-income households from health-damaging housing conditions, but only relates to conditions inside the front door. Indeed, there has been concern about investing public resources in bringing individual dwellings up to the decent homes standard when the neighbourhood is problematic and threatens demand for the renovated homes because people do not want to live there. This led to a third revision of the implementation guidance for local authorities and housing organisations to incorporate provision for not bringing homes up to the standard if they are in low-demand areas that are better scheduled for redevelopment (ODPM, 2004).

Clearly, the possibility of neighbourhood blight is considerable in circumstances where redevelopment is being contemplated, given the long lead-in times for redevelopment schemes. This requires both preventative and ameliorative strategies. In Liverpool, short-term NR funding is being used to arrest further physical deterioration and consult with remaining residents in areas most affected by low housing demand (Yoh, undated). The aim is to support these areas until long-term solutions and funding are identified through the HMR initiative. In England, The Housing Corporation's *Toolkit of Sustainability Indicators* is one of the resources available to social housing landlords to guide the development of data analyses to inform decisions about housing investment (Long, 2001). Nine factors are identified: demand for housing; reputation or image of the community; crime and antisocial behaviour; social exclusion and poverty; the accessibility of employment, facilities and services; the quality of the built and green environment; the quality, design and layout of housing; the extent of social cohesion; and the social mix of the community. Analyses of indicators based on these factors are used to assess the risk involved in making investments to improve housing in particularly problematic areas. This can lead to some of the worst areas with some of the most vulnerable tenants being assessed as very risky investments, reinforcing the need to support these areas until major regeneration programmes can be developed and delivered.

The central issue in this respect is that many neighbourhoods require more than decent homes investment to ensure their long-term sustainability as places where people want to live. How decent homes and decent neighbourhoods articulate together was considered by the UK Parliament's Housing, Planning, Local Government and the Regions Committee in 2004 (ODPM/Housing, Planning, Local Government and the Regions Committee, 2004). Along with recommendations for improving the decent homes standard as it applies to individual dwellings, the Committee recommended that a dwelling should only meet the decency standard if the external environment is also 'decent and sustainable' (para 87). This recommendation was rejected by the government with the rather nebulous reasoning that it had already recognised that meeting the decent homes standard should be addressed within a wider regeneration context.

Research on the impact of neighbourhood conditions on residents' health could, of course, be a start for defining a 'decent neighbourhoods' standard. Over 10 years ago Macintyre et al (1993) argued that research about neighbourhood effects on health needed to focus on actual neighbourhood attributes rather than essentially surrogate measures such as SES. Discriminating between neighbourhood characteristics and their effects on different health outcomes could also help to inform the development and prioritisation of intervention measures. Although there is a danger of reductionism and failure to appreciate the complexity and dynamics of health as an emergent property with this approach, there may be some attributes that justify intervention as a single issue. Introducing trees and integrated greenery into residential environments is one example, deserving a much higher profile in public health than currently (see below).

There is also a cluster of attributes that can be described as liveability. The concept derives from what residents say matters to them, summarised in the following passage from a recent MORI report:

> When we specifically look at how people describe their local area we can see, both in terms of positive and negative associations, that similar points come out time and again. Most frequently, words and phrases relating to the cleanliness and safety of the area are top of mind with a general desire for a more *friendly, clean and safe place* with *no litter or graffiti.* Issues relating to *green space* are also widely mentioned. (Collinge et al, 2005, p 20; emphasis added)

The MORI research reports that perceptions of liveability in England have been improving recently, after a long period of decline. Although visible problems are the main manifestation, such as litter, rubbish, graffiti, vandal damage, dumped cars or scruffy gardens, related issues are the incidence of burglary and robbery, activities for teenagers and facilities for young children. The visible aspect can be regarded as an emergent property, with underlying attributes likely to include child or teenager densities, the quality of services and amenities, and the character of the physical environment, particularly negative effects on area satisfaction of increasing proportions of either high-rise or terraced housing (Collinge et al, 2005). Another relevant attribute, from the US evidence, might be the presence or absence of more affluent households, or good neighbourhood management.

Liveability encompasses neighbourhood attributes that have been found to correlate with health outcomes independently of individual characteristics. These include amounts of integrated greenspace and trees, relationships with neighbours, the level of vandalised property and serious littering, and perceived levels of crime and safety (Blackman and Harvey, 2001; Weich et al, 2001; de Vries et al, 2003; Saelens et al, 2003; Wen et al, 2003; Cho et al, 2005). Among some of the most intriguing evidence is the range of possible benefits to health that appears to be associated with trees and greenery.

Studies carried out by Frances Kuo and William Sullivan in low-income neighbourhoods of Chicago have found fewer incivilities, less violence and aggression, and lower fear of crime as amounts of trees and greenery in the immediate residential environment increase (Kuo and Sullivan, 2001a). The mitigation of aggression has been linked to a restorative effect of greenery and contact with nature, especially when mental fatigue occurs because an environment makes heavy attentional demands, or coping is disadvantaged by poverty or an impairment (Kuo and Sullivan, 2001b). A study by de Vries et al (2003), based on neighbourhoods of around 1,500 people in the Netherlands, found that a 10% increase in the amount of greenspace was associated with a decline in the number of self-reported symptoms of ill-health equivalent to being five years younger. In greener environments, people reported fewer symptoms and had better self-reported general and mental health.

An important potential contribution of neighbourhoods to health is to encourage outdoor exercise, but this is less likely in neighbourhoods that are unattractive, unsafe or where there is nowhere to walk to, such as local shops or a park. Ellaway et al (2005) explored this issue with an analysis of survey data for adults living in eight European cities from the WHO LARES study. They found that living in residential environments with high levels of greenery tripled the odds of frequent physical activity among respondents, controlling for respondents' age, gender, SES and city of residence. Using a body mass index (BMI) calculation from self-reported heights and weights, they also found that the effect on physical activity was reflected in lower levels of being overweight or obese among respondents living in neighbourhoods with a lot of greenery. There was an additional effect for a measure of incivilities based on surveyors' reports of levels of graffiti, litter and dog mess. In residential environments with high levels of incivilities, the likelihood of being more physically active was reduced by almost 50% and the likelihood of being overweight or obese increased by about 50%.

Vegetation is often regarded as contributing to fear of crime because of the cover it provides for criminal activities. However, this seems to be an issue about the type of greenery, especially if it is dense and restricts visibility. Greenery that maintains visibility with widely spaced trees with high canopies and low-growing shrubs and flower beds is likely to bring significant health benefits and minimise any perceived risk. The evidence points to a dose–response relationship between the amount of exposure to trees and greenery and these beneficial effects, although even a low dose of a few trees and grass has been shown to correlate with reduced aggressive behaviour, better management of major life issues by residents and neighbourhood social ties (Kuo and Sullivan, 2001b). Police reports of both property crimes and violent crimes have been found to reduce the greener the surroundings of inner-city apartment buildings (Kuo and Sullivan, 2001a).

Neighbourhoods with green common spaces and trees compared to relatively barren common spaces have been linked with more outdoor activity and sociability (Sullivan et al, 2004). Trees and grass appear to support the common use of outdoor space and promote informal social contact, as well as promoting a sense of safety and feeling part of the neighbourhood (Kuo et al, 1998). Spaces with trees have also been found to attract more mixed groups of young people and adults compared to treeless spaces (Coley et al, 1997). Natural elements such as trees appear to promote social interactions, the monitoring of outdoor areas and the supervision of children.

Two further studies, by Taylor et al (2001, 2002), follow up the possible benefits of greenery for children. Attentional functioning was found to improve after activities in green settings, and symptoms associated with Attention Deficit/Hyperactivity Disorder (ADHD) declined the 'greener' a child's play area. Girls living in high-rise flats were found to have better concentration and self-discipline the better the view of natural surroundings from their homes, with an effect on boys absent possibly because of less time spent playing at home. An earlier study by Taylor et al (1998) found that levels of play and access to adults among children were much lower in relatively barren, low-vegetation surroundings compared to high vegetation spaces around urban social housing.

Several studies have identified a relationship between living in high-rise flats and behavioural and respiratory problems among children, linking this to social isolation and restricted play activities. Wells (2000), however, suggests that disconnection from nature could explain much of this effect. She argues that it is the restorative effects of natural surroundings that children living in high-rise flats are denied, and tested this in a small longitudinal study of low-income urban families that were moved from poor to better housing. Children who experienced the greatest increase in the naturalness of their home environment following their move also scored markedly better than other children on a measure of cognitive functioning used to assess ADHD, controlling for their pre-move score.

The importance of a connection with nature is also supported by the Kaplans' work on the psychological benefits of natural environment experiences, and studies such as Roger Ulrich's work linking faster recovery from surgery with natural views from the hospital room (Ulrich, 1984; Kaplan and Kaplan, 1989). Most of the studies of the effects of neighbourhood greenery on health and behaviour are from the US but there is also some European evidence. Overall, the evidence strongly points to the importance to human health and well-being of incorporating trees and greenery into residential settings, as well as means to access them visually and physically. The type of greenery appears to matter: not so dense as to cause concerns about personal safety but also not homogeneous grassed areas. Native plantings of high-canopy trees and low shrubs and flower borders, attracting wildlife and environmentally beneficial, are advocated by Jackson (2003).

Evidence about the beneficial effects of neighbourhood trees and greenery is strong, but an important argument of this book is that single-cause explanations are rarely the whole picture. It is important, therefore, to consider the causal combinations that make places not simply the sum of their parts, their residents and their environments, but people–environment systems with emergent properties.

Causal combinations and the emergence of neighbourhoods

Galea et al (2005) provide an example of how this complexity works in their study of drug misuse. They identify four 'primary determinants' of drug-use risk behaviour: neighbourhood deprivation, residential segregation, income distribution and population density. These primary determinants, they suggest, have four secondary consequences which, if present, may mediate the relationship between the primary determinants and drug misuse. These are the built environment, access to substances, the availability of public transport, and social and health services. In addition to these primary and secondary determinants, their model includes individual-level characteristics that may also be influenced by the wider environment and play a mediating or moderating role. These include family history, individual SES, social networks and support, and levels of individual stress.

Galea et al cite a wide range of studies with supporting evidence about the significance of these influences on drug misuse, although they recognise that complex interactions are likely to be involved, which mean that any neighbourhood effect is likely to be contingent on other conditions and vary according to how they combine in any particular instance. Underlying most of these influences is the increased likelihood of risky drug use if people are exposed to life stressors such as criminal victimisation or worklessness, or chronic social strain caused by frustrated aspirations, discrimination or threatening environments. Given that these conditions tend to cluster in places, these places create a receptive context for drug dealers and positive feedback sets in as residents have greater exposure to opportunities to obtain drugs. A degree of tolerance may then occur among the community, which is compounded by a lack of alternative opportunities or pleasures in life. Neighbourhood disadvantage increases the likelihood of drug problems but does not determine that these problems will take root or affect more than a minority of people in a disadvantaged neighbourhood. Kadushin et al (1998) refer to a 'substance use system' in which there is a dynamic interplay between the physical and social environments and substance use and misuse. Their analysis of survey data on substance use found that, even after individual characteristics were controlled for, qualities of both people's physical and interpersonal environments were strongly associated with substance dependency. While these environments do not determine this outcome, their findings suggest that bringing about change in drug and alcohol use without fundamentally changing the environments where use takes place is an uphill task. Hembree et al (2005), for instance, single out deterioration of the built environment as associated with an increased likelihood of fatal accidental drug overdose, and Jacobson (2004) identifies places as having a role in rates of attrition from substance abuse programmes in the US. He suggests that a 'treatment ecology' exists whereby neighbourhood disadvantage, drug availability, community resources, restorative qualities of the neighbourhood and travel burden affect the chances of successful treatment outcomes.

Wilson et al (2005) found among a sample of middle-school students that as their respondents reported more problems of neighbourhood disorder and a lower sense of hope, they were more likely to report using alcohol, tobacco and marijuana. They argue that their results point to a need to emphasise creating safer neighbourhoods that support the development of a stronger sense of hope for the future.

Both neighbourhood deprivation and residential instability appear to be important in influencing rates of drug activity (Freisthler et al, 2005). Boardman et al (2001) found in their study of neighbourhoods in Detroit that neighbourhood disadvantage was at least as important as individual-level education and income in explaining adult drug-related behaviours. There was also an interaction with income, such that the association between neighbourhood disadvantage and drug use was stronger among adults in low-income families. Those on higher incomes, but living in generally low-income neighbourhoods, appeared to be relatively immune to this effect.

Stafford and Marmot (2003) also find evidence from the Whitehall II study of civil servants in London that the general and mental health of respondents in lower-status jobs was more affected by living in deprived neighbourhoods than those in higher-status jobs. Further evidence of this interaction comes from a study by Kobetz et al (2003), which found that neighbourhood poverty had a stronger effect on the health of women if their income was below the neighbourhood median. However, Parkes and Kearns (2006), in their analysis of a large Scottish survey dataset, found that the health of more affluent home owners was more likely than low-income social housing tenants to be affected by poor neighbourhood conditions. They suggest that this may be due to more pessimistic expectations among social housing tenants, with a greater acceptance of deviant behaviour, while home owners expect fewer neighbourhood problems, which then have more impact when they do occur. This did not hold, however, for walking, where people with low incomes, as indicated by non-car ownership, were more likely to walk for fitness or pleasure if they liked the appearance of their neighbourhood.

Gender is another factor in considering interaction effects. Ellaway and Macintyre (2001) report results showing a stronger effect of neighbourhood problems and cohesion on the symptomatic health of women than men. Parkes and Kearns (2006) found that women who had experienced crime were more likely than men who had experienced crime to make frequent GP visits, possibly reflecting a greater sense of vulnerability. They also found that older people's health was more affected than younger people by disputes, lack of neighbourly help and high levels of neighbourhood problems.

The 'neighbourhood effect' seems better thought of as a set of relationships between environmental press spanning social attributes, physical attributes and facilities/services, and individuals with their own attributes and household contexts. As Figure 3.2 indicated, these relationships engender adaptive behaviours, which have outcomes with consequences for individual health status, but which also create collective variables that feed back to influence individual behaviour and health. Of considerable significance in this respect appears to be whether there is a feeling of belonging to the neighbourhood.

Popay et al (2003) explore how neighbourhood conditions interact with individuals' normative values. They found that in deprived areas many more residents than in wealthier areas were unhappy with living in the neighbourhood and felt that they did not belong or wanted to leave. The contrast in perceptions about whether the neighbourhood was a good place to bring up children was particularly stark. Between 40% and 60% of residents in the deprived areas considered that this was not the case, compared with just 4%-6% in the advantaged areas. However, differences between socioeconomically similar areas were sometimes as great as or greater than those between contrasting areas. Popay et al see this as a problem of dissonance between what residents value and what they experience. This was especially marked in one of the deprived areas that had undergone a rapid decline and had acquired a stigma that was possibly intensified by being targeted for regeneration. There was also a strong individual dimension. Respondents in the same area could express very different levels of dissonance depending on their sense of belonging to the area and relationships with nearby family or friends. High dissonance, Popay et al suggest, is a cause of health problems, both directly and indirectly through the behaviour it induces. A graphic quote from one of their interviewees, a lone parent feeling trapped and isolated living in an 'improper place', and who had seen her weight increase from 10 to 15 stones over 18 months, illustrates the possible effect:

> The doctor put me on Prozac a few months back for living here. Because it's depressing. You get up, you look around and all you see is junkies ... I know one day I will come off, I will get off here. I mean I started drinking a hell of a lot more since I've been on here. I drink every night. I have a drink every night just to get to sleep. I smoke more as well. There's a lot of things. (Popay et al, 2003, p 68)

Popay et al argue that people respond to dissonance: they may take action to deal with problems or move house, or – what they commonly found – keep themselves to themselves, possibly turning to drinking and smoking. They suggest that the extent of this last coping strategy, what they call a 'privatisation of everyday life', is likely to make some neighbourhoods unreceptive contexts for renewal programmes.

Kuo and Sullivan (2001b) identify a link between poor liveability and conflict behaviour in their study of a Chicago social housing scheme. They believe that this link operates through a pathway of *attentional fatigue* caused by excessive environment press in disadvantaged neighbourhoods and its effects on inattentiveness, irritability and impulsiveness. Deprived neighbourhoods are more likely to make attentional demands due to fear of crime, noise, traffic or crowding. If these demands to pay attention or concentrate are not relieved then aggressive or violent behaviour is more likely, especially if poverty brings added susceptibility and vulnerability. Kuo and Sullivan investigated the role of restorative contact with greenery and nature in the residential environment and found that forms of aggression such as threatening behaviour or throwing objects were less likely among residents living near trees and greenery compared to residents whose immediate surroundings had little or no vegetation. This did not, however, extend to more violent forms of aggression or aggression towards children. They argue that this relationship is best explained by the restorative effects of greenery.

Conclusion: neighbourhoods and policy

It is not just neighbourhoods that introduce place effects into the relationship between individual socioeconomic level and health outcomes. Workplaces have also been found to have an effect, with the association between individual SES and health outcomes varying by place of work and with different consequences for men and women (Vahtera et al, 1999). Occupational factors seem to be more important for men's health than for women's health, with the home environment exercising a stronger influence among women (Stafford et al, 2005). Similar mechanisms may be involved, especially control (at home or work) and an imbalance between effort and reward, with these affecting both mental and physical health.

The influence of neighbourhood conditions on health, therefore, should be considered in the context of other influences, and this can point to some possible common causes. A study based on the Oxford Healthy Life Survey by Evans et al (2000) compares the effects on health of different housing and neighbourhood problems with the effects of demographic, psychosocial, work and lifestyle factors. This was a cross-sectional multivariable analysis of a large sample of adults of working age. The most important factors found to be most consistently associated with poorer self-reported health were worklessness, worry about pressure at work, worry about money, cold housing, being female, and not taking enough vigorous physical exercise. Respondents who reported being unable to keep their home warm enough in winter were significantly more likely to have asthma or a long-standing illness generally, and made double the number of visits to the GP's surgery and to outpatient departments than other respondents. This effect of cold housing was greater than that of smoking, not taking vigorous exercise or drinking alcohol. Of generally at least equal importance to cold housing, however, were two 'worry variables': worry about pressure at work and worry about money.

Regarding neighbourhood conditions specifically, Evans et al found that health was affected by poor public transport, smells and fumes, noise, lack of open spaces and vandalism, but none of these neighbourhood variables exceeded the marked effects on health of worklessness, worry about pressure at work or about money, and cold housing. However, their analysis is quite limited in exploring neighbourhood problems. For example, a marked association between wanting to move from the local area and poorer mental health and social functioning is apparent in one of the tables in their article but is not commented on in the article. In addition, while 15% of respondents wanted to move area, just 8% reported a cold home. Nevertheless, worries about pressure at work and money affected a fifth and a quarter of respondents respectively, and were overall more strongly associated with poor health than neighbourhood or lifestyle variables. There are, though, many reasons why people worry. While work and money may often be more of a worry than home and neighbourhood, the latter can clearly be troubling and stressful, cause dissonance and attentional fatigue, and reflect on our sense of control and self-esteem (Wen et al, 2005).

Many studies have documented an association between both contextual and compositional neighbourhood characteristics and individual health outcomes, but these effects do appear to be weak compared to individual characteristics and their influence on health. There are, however, theoretical reasons for questioning whether an 'independent' neighbourhood effect can be regarded as 'real'. The techniques that are used in statistical studies of neighbourhood effects separate out two sources of variation. The first is that associated with aggregate spatial data, treating neighbourhoods as cases that structure outcomes for individuals living in these neighbourhoods depending on variation in neighbourhood type. The second is that associated with data for individuals, treating individuals as cases whose characteristics also display structured patterns that are mirrored in structured outcomes. Yet the neighbourhood data used are often not data on neighbourhood cases but individual data aggregated into neighbourhood units. Not only could this be measuring the same thing in different ways, with the demonstration of separate effects possibly no more than an artefact of the statistical techniques used, but it ignores the fact that there are no social or economic characteristics of places that can exist separately from individuals. As Lawton argued, all parts of the local situation enter the situation as participants.

A single variable having an independent effect is probably rare in the real world, although *sufficiency* can be a feature of causal combinations, such as the apparently sufficient effect of worklessness in raising smoking prevalence to very high levels among people in this condition (discussed in Chapter Two). Sufficiency exists when a condition on its own is capable of producing an outcome (Ragin, 2000). Generally, however, the outcomes of interest in neighbourhood renewal and health are much more likely to have complex causations and to owe their existence to causal combinations. Conventional multivariable models explore causal complexity by investigating interaction effects. For example, de Vries et al (2003) found that the effect of living in a green environment on health was stronger among people with a lower level of education, homecarers and older people than other groups. This might be because these groups interact with the local environment more often, experience a higher health gain from greenery than better-off and more healthy people (a ceiling effect), or adopt a more active lifestyle in greener neighbourhoods.

Another example of interaction is the study by Stafford et al (2005), which found that all of the between-neighbourhood variation in self-reported health among men could be explained by economic level and family type, but these variables only explained 41% of the between-neighbourhood variation among women. All the variation was explained for women, however, when variables measuring aspects of social capital, provision of amenities and the physical environment were added to the model. These features of the neighbourhood had an effect on women's health that was absent for men, suggesting both a greater vulnerability among women to these effects and a greater potential for women to benefit from measures to improve social cohesion and poor-quality environments.

An interaction with gender means that causal combinations with one gender produce a different outcome to causal combinations with the other gender. Ragin's (2000) method of QCA is a better way of exploring this than conventional multivariate models, although the latter do have a role in theory testing. QCA also focuses our attention on outcomes as space–time states rather than on continuous variation in a dependent variable. It is therefore much more suited to exploring how to achieve policy outcomes because the concern is with the condition of cases, in terms of current and possible future states, rather than the abstract notion of variation in a variable.

Interactions produce phenomena beyond individuals: this is modelled very transparently in QCA by looking at the causal combinations associated with an outcome. Rather than attempt to capture these scales by rather artificially separating variation into levels, as with multi-level models, QCA tabulations can include attributes believed to represent key parameter values, possibly at different system levels, that affect outcomes for the cases being examined. This selection should be made on theoretical grounds rather than simply data mining. For example, a QCA model of a health outcome could include gender or worklessness as individual system attributes, liveability or social capital as neighbourhood system attributes, and employment rate or health care spending as regional system attributes. Using a 'higher-level' system attribute can help with interpretation by limiting the number of attributes under consideration. Liveability, for example, might be a composite index comprised of several neighbourhood problems as reported by individual residents.

QCA requires states to be defined. In other words, we need to define 'good' and 'bad' liveability, a 'lot' or 'little' greenery, and so on. We are in fact then working with terms that relate well to policy and performance management, and specifically to *targets*, an issue explored in the next chapter. These distinctions involve judgements, whether from user or public consultation, professional judgement or statistical thresholds, guided by theory. Working with *states* rather than continuums requires an explicitness that is not only helpful methodologically but also politically. What, for example, is a 'decent neighbourhood', as opposed to a neighbourhood that relative to another one is 20% more deprived?

The neighbourhood system is the walkable, experiential zone centred on the domestic home setting, up a level from the household system. Up a scale from the neighbourhood is the travel-to-work area or 'city region', and up a further level is the phase space defined by economic and welfare regimes. This last level is one of variation in key upstream control parameters. Health is likely to be affected at all levels but in different ways. Across countries, income inequality is associated with mortality in some countries but not others, and this appears to reflect different national-scale policies (Ross et al, 2005). Travel-to-work areas will influence aspects of health affected by the availability of employment, such as limiting illnesses (Sacker et al, 2006). General health, by contrast, may be influenced more by who people live with at the household level. In complexity theory there is no necessary privileging of any level in explanations, and 'downstream' change is recognised as having the potential of causing 'upstream' change as well. Health inequalities demand intervention at all levels. While the neighbourhood level will not be sufficient, it is necessary.

Whether in terms of Popay et al's dissonance, Kuo and Sullivan's attentional fatigue, or Evans et al's worry, neighbourhoods may seem unimportant to health when there is a reasonable equilibrium between where we live and how we want to live. But if these move far from equilibrium then we may (mal)adapt in ways that affect our health and possibly damage it. A better concept than equilibrium, however, is Lawton's concept of dynamic adaptability to environment press. We look for stimulation and feedback from environments – some *press* and *buoying* – and not blandness. As long as environment press is within a tolerable range we enjoy a dynamic balance between our needs for autonomy and participation, and the opportunities for autonomy and participation afforded by our living environments.

FIVE

Neighbourhood renewal and health inequalities

Lupton (2003, p 1) comments that, 'Rarely has the neighbourhood enjoyed as high a profile in public policy as it does today'. She continues with a list of the many area-based initiatives (ABIs) introduced by Labour governments since 1997. In England, the focus on neighbourhoods in strategies to tackle deprivation has mainly been concerned with improving the delivery of public services in deprived areas so as to achieve measurable improvements in key outcomes across health, employment, education, housing and crime. Similar approaches exist in Scotland, Wales and Northern Ireland, but currently with less emphasis on performance assessment and management. While there are substantial additional resources for these programmes, they also emphasise news ways of working that promote partnerships and community engagement.

Neighbourhood renewal: its targets and performance

England's National Strategy for Neighbourhood Renewal was launched in 2001. It is one of the most significant of a wide range of social policy initiatives launched by the New Labour government after the Conservatives were defeated in 1997, and which has included both ABIs and national programmes such as the drive to eliminate child poverty (HM Treasury, 2005). The programme was shaped by a series of reports from 18 Policy Action Teams, which concluded that past initiatives had failed sufficiently to tackle the problems of depressed local economies and the safety and stability of local communities, or to improve public services for the most disadvantaged residents and involve residents in decisions affecting them (SEU, 2001). They also crucially lacked effective local leadership, partnership working and information.

These last issues reflect the wider shift in public policy that has been occurring under New Labour, and indeed began earlier in the 1990s under the Conservatives. This has been away from *government* through blueprint and direct service delivery dominated by public sector professionals, and towards *governance* through networks that bring different public, private and voluntary/community actors together to agree, plan and deliver programmes that often cross organisational boundaries (Stoker, 1998; Kooiman, 2003). This is an agenda that is very much about achieving the delivery of measurable outcomes (hence the emphasis on information), but not prescribing in detail organisational arrangements on the ground. The emphasis is on working differently, and tackling joined-up problems with joined-up solutions (Cabinet Office, 1999). Local actors are given space and incentives to realise the policy intent from the centre by developing the concrete organisational arrangements locally. Harrison and Wood (1999) call this 'manipulated emergence' to distinguish it from the tighter policy–action regime that marked an earlier post-war era in British public policy characterised more by technocratic blueprints.

The emphasis on how social problems are interlinked is not new and characterised earlier urban policy initiatives (Blackman, 1995; Atkinson et al, 2006). The concern with delivery, however, is a new emphasis, particularly performance management from the centre. This has introduced a tension between national government prescription of both targets and partnerships, which it then holds to account for delivery, and local autonomy to decide on priorities (Newman, 2001; Peckham et al, 2005). The new governance agenda has framed a role for elected local authorities as 'community leaders' working together with partners on the well-being of their communities. The NR strategy, however, is delivered not through local government but through LSPs accountable to regional offices of national government. Indeed it, like the related New Deal for Communities programme, was influenced by the Commission on Social Justice set up by the Labour Party when in opposition, which argued against channelling programmes through local authorities (Commission on Social Justice, 1994). They were seen as often poor at involving and responding to the needs of disadvantaged communities. The pendulum is swinging back to recognising the lead democratic and strategic role of the local authority, and while there is little sign of the audit culture waning, there is growing pressure to reduce further the scale and complexity of national targets and inspection, and allow more local variation in outcomes (Lyons, 2006). It will be interesting to see how this unfolds, and whether the current range of health inequality targets remain intact.

The location of the NR strategy within an audit regime makes it a different initiative to past urban programmes. In urban policy this culture has evolved from measuring project-based outputs in the 1980s and 1990s, to topics such as health, crime and worklessness representing domains of comprehensive programmes with their own outcome-based targets (Atkinson et al, 2006).The national targets are prescriptive, but there is also an expectation that local targets are developed alongside them. While the rationale for targets is that the considerable extra public spending on these programmes needs to achieve demonstrable improvements, how they are to be delivered is prescribed very little. Scope is left for local approaches to be developed, but this has raised issues about whether targets are achievable with the means available. This connection between targets and means is left fairly vague, with resulting difficulties in distinguishing between the effects of local circumstances on the one hand and of national policy intent on the other (Peckham and Exworthy, 2003; Millward, 2005).

The performance management framework for the NR strategy and indeed all major public services and social programmes in England is based on Public Service Agreements (PSAs) and 'floor targets'. PSAs were introduced by the new Labour government following its first 'comprehensive spending review' in 1998.They are a Treasury method of tying government departments into agreements to deliver measurable results in exchange for additional public spending. Departments have to report progress against their targets in annual reports. PSAs have been developed in subsequent spending reviews, including focusing down on fewer key priorities and outcomes, and supplementing these with lower-level input targets and milestones that should underpin delivery against the PSA targets. These cascade down to local government, where achievement of local PSA targets attracts additional funding, and to the local NHS and LSPs, whose funding allocations are conditional on satisfactory performance against targets. Some targets are shared between services and between national and local government, including health targets.

In 2000, a specific type of target was introduced for monitoring progress with tackling deprivation called a 'floor target'. These are innovative inequality targets aimed at 'levering up' the performance of public services in deprived areas so that outcomes move towards national averages.They span education, employment, enterprise, crime, housing, liveability, health, road accidents and regional economic growth, and monitor progress in terms of either the inequality gap or a target minimum level of performance. They are 'owned' by the appropriate government departments, and some are jointly owned. The floor targets for health are owned by the Department of Health and target inequalities in death rates from circulatory illnesses, cancer and suicide, life expectancy and smoking, and rates of infant mortality, teenage conceptions and childhood obesity.The reduction in teenage conceptions is a joint target with the Department for Education and

Skills, and the obesity target is a joint target with the Department for Education and Skills and the Department for Culture, Media and Sport. It is of course recognised that other outcome areas such as improvements in employment and housing will make important contributions to the health targets.

Liveability became an additional focus following the 2004 Public Spending Review, which introduced a new target for local authorities, the police and other partners to 'improve liveability and strengthen communities' (HM Treasury, 2004, p 65). The aspiration of better service delivery at neighbourhood level is now complemented by this aim of 'cleaner, safer, greener' neighbourhoods. Progress will be monitored using local survey data.

The Neighbourhood Renewal Unit (NRU) in the ODPM has had particular responsibility for securing delivery of floor targets against the six key outcome areas for the NR Strategy of health, worklessness, crime, education, housing and liveability. In May 2006, the ODPM was reorganised as the Department for Communities and Local Government, and the NRU was incorporated into the Department's new Places and Communities Group. Among the Group's responsibilites are LSPs, LAAs and the Neighbourhood Renewal Fund (NRF). The NRF was established as a short-term fund to help achieve the NR floor targets but has been extended twice since its inception in 2001.

The first allocation was £800 million over three years among 88 local authority areas scoring poorly on the official Indices of Deprivation. The most recent allocation is £1.05 billion over the two years from 2006/07 among 86 local authority areas. NRF for six areas is being phased out, reflecting the government's evaluation that enough progress has been made in these areas and that they do not need extra resources on top of the mainstream budgets of their local public services. Three further local authority areas were added to those eligible for NRF and, in addition, a new £265 million Safer Stronger Communities Fund has been introduced with a 'neighbourhood element' targeted at 84 local authorities that contain pockets of deprivation in small neighbourhoods. A 'cleaner, safer, greener' element of the Safer Stronger Communities Fund is targeted at 50 of these authorities so that they can also make improvements to their public spaces.

Life expectancy is an example of how general PSA targets have been combined with floor targets to narrow inequality. The Department of Health has a target of improving the health of the general population by increasing male life expectancy to 78.6 years and female life expectancy to 82.5 years by 2010. To help achieve this, the 2010 PSA target for heart disease and stroke is to reduce these mortality rates among the under-75s by at least 40%. It is possible that such a target could be achieved while inequalities increase, but this would mean that the Department of Health misses its floor target. This is for at least a 40% reduction in the inequalities gap between the fifth of areas with the worst health and deprivation indicators and the population as a whole (see, however, the discussion in Chapter One about the confusion regarding absolute and relative differences in formulating these targets). This introduction of 'floor' elements to PSA targets is a device that is meant to narrow inequalities during a period when incomes, health and other quality-of-life measures are improving generally. This situation risks deprived areas and groups failing to improve at the same rate and falling further behind. In health, the baseline comparator of the lowest quintile of areas as ranked by the Indices of Deprivation has also been replaced by the bottom quintile on a new health-weighted index, with local authorities, PCTs and LSPs in these areas belonging to the Spearhead Group, with responsibility for making faster overall progress against the floor targets. These local organisations are therefore the delivery agents for meeting the 'floor' element of PSA targets.

In April 2005, most floor targets were grouped under one of six key outcome areas: health, education, crime, worklessness, housing and liveability. The current floor targets can be found at www.neighbourhood.gov.uk, where the 'floor targets interactive' system also allows progress towards the targets to be monitored, compared and displayed as tables and graphs. A summary is presented in Table 5.1.

Table 5.1 shows that so far there has been a narrowing in gaps across four of the key themes of the NR strategy: employment, education, crime and housing. Housing conditions in NRF areas have improved markedly as a result of the considerable input of resources to the social housing system to bring the stock up to the decent homes standard. Improvements in education also reflect significant additional spending as well as tighter performance management. Crime has fallen in NRF areas but the level of crime remains high compared to other parts of the country. Liveability is a relatively new floor target, so progress cannot be evaluated at this stage but the signs are quite encouraging (see Chapter Four).

There are certainly no signs of a general transformation of conditions in the NRF areas, although it is early days yet. Some areas have achieved impressive results but others have struggled to improve their position

Table 5.1: The Neighbourhood Renewal Strategy floor targets: progress up to 2004

Floor target	Indicators	Progress to date
Employment rate	Over the 3 years to spring 2008, increase the employment rate, and reduce the differences in the overall rate and the rates for disadvantaged groups (lone parents, ethnic minorities, people aged 50 and over, those with the lowest qualifications), and those living in the local authority wards with the poorest initial labour market position.	The overall English employment rate rose from 73.3% in 1997 to 74.8% in 2004, and for NRF areas from 67.2% to 69.5%, closing the gap slightly from 6.1% to 5.3%. Between 2001 and 2004, the employment rate gap for lone parents, people aged 50 and over, and those with the lowest qualifications narrowed slightly, but for ethnic minorities widened slightly.
Education	There are several floor targets for education, with indicators for child development and achievement at ages 11, 14 and 16. The target for age 16 is that, by 2008, 60% of students achieve the equivalent of 5 GCSEs at grades A* to C; and in all schools at least 25% of pupils achieve this standard by 2006, rising to 30% by 2008.	The national GCSE achievement rate increased from 46.3% in 1998 to 53.7% in 2004, and for NRF areas from 36.1% to 46.1%, closing the gap from 10.2% to 7.6%. The school targets are an important focus for individual LSP NR strategies.
Health	Substantially reduce mortality rates by 2010: from heart disease and stroke and related diseases by at least 40% in people under 75, with at least a 40% reduction in the inequalities gap between the fifth of areas with the worst health and deprivation indicators and the population as a whole; from cancer by at least 20% in people under 75, with a reduction in the inequalities gap of at least 6% between the fifth of areas with the worst health and deprivation indicators and the population as a whole.	There is a continuing widening of inequalities in life expectancy and infant mortality, but evidence of a narrowing of the gap in premature deaths from circulatory diseases and, to a lesser extent, cancers. The national prevalence of smoking fell between 1998 and 2003 but the gap between manual and other groups did not narrow.

Table 5.1: contd.../

Floor target	Indicators	Progress to date
Health contd.../	Reduce health inequalities by 10% by 2010 as measured by infant mortality and life expectancy at birth.	The national teenage conceptions rate (per 1,000 females aged 15-17) fell from 46.0 in 1996-98 (3-year rolling average) to 42.4 in 2001-03, and in NRF areas from 58.7 to 54.1, closing the gap slightly from 12.7% to 11.7%.
	Tackle the underlying determinants of ill-health and health inequalities by reducing adult smoking rates to 21% or less by 2010, with a reduction in prevalence among routine and manual groups to 26% or less.	
	Reduce the under-18 conception rate by 50% by 2010 as part of a broader strategy to improve sexual health.	
Crime	Reduce crime by 15%, and further in high crime areas, by 2007-08.	The national overall crime rate fell from 69.3 in 2003 (reported crimes per 1,000 population) to 64.0 in 2004, and in NRF areas from 90.9 to 82.6, closing the gap slightly from 21.6% to 18.6%.
		Nationally, burglary rates fell from 20.8 in 1999 to 14.7 in 2004, and from 30.6 to 20.7 in NRF areas.
Housing	By 2010, bring all social housing into a decent condition with most of this improvement taking place in deprived areas, and for vulnerable households in the private sector, including families with children, increase the proportion who live in homes that are in decent condition.	Housing conditions across NRF areas have improved steadily with the number of non-decent social sector homes falling by 38% since 1996 (from 1.4m to 0.8m). However, high levels of non-decent housing continue to be more prevalent in areas where there are local concentrations of deprivation.
Liveability	Lead the delivery of cleaner, safer and greener public spaces and improvement of the quality of the built environment in deprived areas and across the country, with measurable improvement by 2008.	Baseline data shows that in 2003/04 23% of local authorities in England and 33% of NRF local authorities had 'unacceptable' levels of litter, in excess of the national baseline. The target is 17% of NRF local authorities by 2008.

Table 5.2: Floor target changes from baseline year to latest year

	Range across top and bottom 5 NRF areas by degree of change							
	Top		5th top		5th from bottom		Bottom	
Floor target	Base	Change	Base	Change	Base	Change	Base	Change
Employment rate (%), 1997-2004	60.2	+14.0	69.0	+9.3	75.2	−3.6	77.2	−8.4
5+ GCSE A*-Cs (%), 1998-2005	39.6	+25.7	22.9	+21.5	42.3	+3.3	37.4	−0.7
Male life expectancy (yrs), 1997-2003	75.5	+5.3	72.2	+3.0	74.2	+0.8	74.2	+0.3
Female life expectancy (yrs), 1997-2003	81.4	+4.4	80.6	+2.1	81.1	−0.1	79.2	−0.6
Teenage conceptions per 1,000, 1999-2003	68.3	−15.8	54.3	−10.9	70.2	+6.5	61.3	+11.0
Burglaries per 1,000 households, 1999-2005	51.1	−27.1	48.2	−24.6	22.8	−0.2	12.6	+1.6

Source: http://www.fti.neighbourhood.gov.uk/

or have even moved backwards. Table 5.2 compares the top and bottom five performing NRF areas for six floor targets, showing how wide this performance is. The figures exclude the proportion of decent homes because complete local data are not available (Table 5.1 uses national survey data). The poor performance with improving life expectancy stands out. This is an outcome that would be expected to take time to show any improvement but it is a cause for concern. The performance assessment of NRF LSPs by regional GOs enables the overall picture to be summarised: 35% have been assessed as making 'good progress', 47% as making 'mixed progress' and 18% are regarded as 'problematic' and needing substantial attention (NRU briefing, November 2005).

The challenge of achieving faster progress than average, which is necessary to achieve the floor targets, is a tough one. A focus for the NRU in assessing progress is comparisons between NRF areas. Figure 5.1 illustrates this with the example of premature deaths from

Figure 5.1: Circulatory diseases premature mortality rate

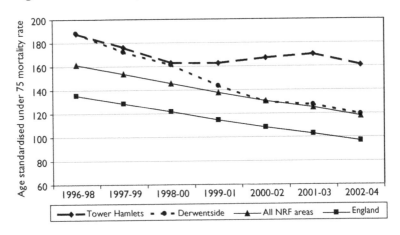

circulatory diseases. There is a marked decline in the English national average since 1996-98, with a slightly sharper decline in the average for all NRF areas. However, when two NRF areas that had similar mortality rates at the start of the period are compared, Derwentside in County Durham and Tower Hamlets in London, a marked difference in their trajectories is evident. These are both very deprived areas. Derwentside, a former coalmining area, has seen its gap with the English average close significantly, paradoxically an effect in part of its loss of health-damaging heavy industry. Tower Hamlets, a multi-ethnic inner London borough, has seen its gap widen. Although the most deprived borough in London, Tower Hamlets is a classic example of wealth and deprivation next door to each other. But it is not just context that explains these differences in performance, as we consider further below.

CHD is more common in lower socioeconomic groups and in certain minority ethnic groups, in particular the South Asian population, than the rest of the population. Tower Hamlets has a large and very deprived Bangladeshi community, which is clearly a factor in explaining the persistence of its high CHD mortality. Generally, the slow progress being made with race equality is a major issue for the NR strategy. Only 59% of the working-age BME population are in work compared to 75% of the working-age population as a whole, a gap of 16% that has not changed much since the early 1980s. Black Caribbean boys are achieving well below average at school compared to white boys, and are three times more likely to be permanently excluded. There are further specific race inequalities regarding health (considered in the next chapter), risk of crime, housing and liveability. Regional GOs are prioritising race equality in the performance management of LSPs, requiring them to demonstrate how they are having a positive impact on their BME populations. The NR strategy is geographically targeted on deprived neighbourhoods, but without improved outcomes for BME groups it will be impossible to meet its targets. Sixty-seven per cent of England's BME population live in the NR areas.

The NR strategy has subsequently been elaborated by other initiatives such as Neighbourhood Management and is taken forward most recently by *Making it Happen in Deprived Neighbourhoods* (ODPM, 2005b). This reviews progress and places more emphasis on improving the performance of existing public services in closing the gap between deprived areas and the rest of the country, as well as tackling inequalities within local authority areas. The latter point is important in that the gap between a local authority's position compared to national averages for key indicators can be substantially due to the problems of particular neighbourhoods within the local authority area. By reducing the gap between these targeted neighbourhoods and the local area average substantial progress can be made with closing the gap between the local authority area average and the national average.

The NR strategy has also influenced governance in England generally with its approach. Devolution of budgets, regulatory powers and decision making to neighbourhood bodies across the country is planned, including more neighbourhood contracts with service providers, and neighbourhood ownership and management of community assets (ODPM, 2005c, 2005d). In part this is driven by a concern about public disengagement from politics and declining turnouts in local elections, especially in the most deprived areas. The liveability agenda is a focus because of its potential to engage people. Burningham and Thrush (2003) make the observation from their study of how disadvantaged groups perceive 'the environment' that 'the environment did not exist as a separate category of concern but was inextricable from broader evaluations of local quality of life and their own sense of agency' (p 533). If people cannot influence what happens in their own surroundings, and if problems with the safety and amenity of these surroundings appear to be beyond the power of local authorities to resolve, then cynicism about democratic government on a wider scale is more likely to follow.

Just as liveability is high up the list of public priorities about what makes a place a good place to live, health services also rank highly (Lyons, 2006). Although extending neighbourhood governance to increase local influence over the commissioning of health care would begin to make devolution of powers to this level look a lot more serious, it is not yet on this agenda.

From targets to causes

Floor targets are a significant innovation in public policy, and an important counterweight to the local variations in health outcomes that would follow from largely devolved decision making about health care and public health. As well as being about reducing inequality on the basis of national comparative measures, they are meant to encourage a focus at the local level on key priorities and on where service improvements and new ways of working are needed. Where the progress being made by an LSP is assessed by its regional GO as not good enough, the GO can intervene to require specific improvement plans to be drawn up, provide additional advisory or consultancy support, or withhold further NRF allocations.

Although only a few years into the NR strategy, by 2004 slow progress was regarded by the ODPM as an issue for many NRF-funded LSPs. For 2004/05 and 2005/06, extra NRF was targeted at the 26 districts with the furthest 'distance to travel' on two or more key targets. This was complemented by the 'Places Project', which involved three areas – Manchester, Nottingham and Southwark – working together to gain a better understanding of the reasons for poor progress against floor target indicators (NRU, 2004). In Nottingham, the process led to a decision to disband and reform the LSP to improve partnership working, which had not been going well and which was regarded as a major obstacle to making more progress. Other problems identified through the Places Project were specific to particular floor targets, such as recruiting and retaining good-quality staff and head teachers in local schools. Poor data for certain indicators was of general significance, with teenage conceptions and other health data at small-area level singled out. A further issue was competing initiatives, targets and reporting arrangements. Underlying many of the problems was believed to be a need for more rigorous analysis, joint planning and performance management at local level. An outcome of the Places Project in this respect, which has been generalised to other LSPs where progress has been an issue, is the use of 'Floor Target Action Plans' as a tool for moving forward with those target areas where performance is some distance below the national floor target.

Floor Target Action Plans are very straightforward in concept and provide a general model for local strategy formulation. They have five main stages. The first is orientation, which means getting the relevant stakeholders together and agreeing on the course of action ('buy-in'). The second is analysis: understanding the situation using data about the nature and extent of problems, their priority, and what is already in place to address them. There is a requirement that the national floor targets are always treated as a priority by NRF-funded LSPs, but they can be supplemented with other local priorities. The third stage is option appraisal, identifying what could be done better or differently. The fourth is agreeing action, adopting plans and putting in place delivery arrangements. The final stage is tracking delivery by setting up arrangements to monitor progress, assess performance and take action to correct underachievement.

Terms such as 'performance' and 'underachievement' run the risk of creating a blame culture, which is not the best environment for learning and improving. How performance management is used is a question of power and how power is exercised and shared. At best, performance management establishes a commonality of purpose, clarity about ownership, accountability for outcomes, and honest and transparent assessments of actual performance, which can include identifying external barriers as well as internal issues. The NR strategy is meant to encourage *joined-up* strategic and improvement planning across each local authority area, and this is now being generalised beyond just NR areas to English local governance as a whole through Community Strategies and LAAs, discussed further below. The key features are being specific about the problems to be tackled and the neighbourhoods and communities being targeted; having plans that deliver improvements in performance, with any risks and issues identified and managed; and establishing both a system and a culture of performance management that maintains a focus on the effectiveness of partnership working and outcomes. Performance management is therefore a framework for communicating and implementing policy and strategy in which *alignment* between strategy and decision making is a central principle. A major challenge for LSPs in this respect is that each partner organisation has its own governance and performance management arrangements, and there is also an expectation that voluntary and community groups participate in processes that can be perceived, if not actually experienced, as managerialist and excluding.

There are different ways in which these issues can be addressed. There needs to be as much integration of existing systems as possible. This includes nesting plans so that there is alignment of purpose and approach between development plans for individuals, through to service delivery plans, departmental and corporate plans, and the Community Strategy. Appropriate styles of working and support for voluntary and community groups are essential. By integrating systems, the aim is that partners are brought together around a common process and concern with understanding and achieving change using shared data. Theory of change thinking is a useful discipline in these circumstances, despite the 'messiness' of what actually occurs in processes of policy formulation and implementation (see Barnes, M. et al, 2005, for an extended discussion of this issue in relation to the HAZ initiative). This is because there does need to be attention paid to the 'black box' that exists between targets on the one hand, and what is being delivered on the ground on the other: that is, the theory of change.

Essentially, there are two stages to this. The first is articulating a theory about the *drivers that engender change* in the outcomes of concern. What is it, for example, that leads to above-average levels of premature mortality in a locality? The second is theories of what interventions will affect these drivers and why these are better than doing something else or nothing at all. Estimates then need to be made of what impact the interventions will have over time, and the resulting trajectory of the outcome measure graphed to show how interventions are planned to close in on the target outcome. Drivers and interventions are likely to overlap between agencies, so a strategic task is to identify the 'golden threads' and win-wins that exist in this respect. For instance, supporting people with drug addiction problems is likely to deliver results across employment, health and crime targets. This justifies a pooling of resources across employment, health and criminal justice agencies, and a focusing of this budget – with its greater critical mass – on those interventions that will have most impact, regardless of the particular delivery organisation.

An example of this approach is as follows, using improved life expectancy as the outcome aimed at. One of the drivers of low life expectancy is high infant mortality among babies whose fathers are in routine and semi-routine occupations. Infant mortality is an outcome of the more prevalent issue of low birth weight, which is strongly related to deprivation (Asthana and Halliday, 2006). The key drivers of low birth weight are smoking during pregnancy, lack of early years support for teenage mothers, lone parenting, low income, problems with accessing good antenatal services, and not breastfeeding. Programmes that address these issues are therefore likely to lower the infant mortality rate and contribute to improving life expectancy, especially if supported by national programmes aimed at improving low incomes.

Teenage conceptions are another driver of infant mortality. They are also a specific health floor target for the NR strategy because teenage conception rates are much higher in the UK than elsewhere in Europe and especially high in deprived areas. Teenagers face higher risks to both themselves and the baby's health compared to pregnancy at a later age, including a 60% higher risk of infant mortality. Halving the number of teenage births would achieve an estimated 10% of the currently targeted reduction in infant mortality rates in England (DH, 2005c). Reducing teenage conceptions is an example of a golden thread where a number of outcomes are possible with successful programmes. These include an impact on the heightened risks of poorer educational and employment outcomes for both mothers and children, the higher rate of dependency on benefits, and the higher incidence of family conflict (Swann et al, 2003). Outcomes for young fathers follow a similar pattern but less is known about teenage fathers.

Performance assessment is about asking whether the theory of change has predicted well. In other words, programmes are put in place because there is a theory that they will work. If the theory is correct the outcome indicators should follow their planned trajectory. Performance management is about taking any necessary corrective action based on one of three possible conclusions if there has been poor prediction. The first is that the intervention was the wrong thing to do to achieve the expected outcome, the second is that it was the right intervention but done wrongly, and the third is that it was the right thing to do, done correctly, but external factors worked against it. This last scenario recognises the importance of context. Taking action if it is the context that is the problem is a question of either moving up a level to change parameters in a larger system (such as introducing new powers of intervention or securing a larger budget), or adjusting the target to recognise the realities of the local context. Context, however, needs to be part of all three possible scenarios: whether an intervention works, or whether a way of delivering an intervention works, are always likely to be context dependent.

The significance of context is also important when it comes to evaluation. Evaluation of the NR strategy has included looking at the similar and contrasting circumstances of LSPs to see if there are general lessons. One such evaluation is the recent report *Improving Floor Target Performance: What Works?* (GFA Consulting, 2005). This reviews progress in the NR areas for three of the key themes: crime, education and worklessness. For each theme, four LSPs that appeared to be making above-average progress were selected as case studies for further investigation. Four attributes emerged as contributing to their success. First, these LSPs worked with a concerted focus that gave collective force to many initiatives aimed at the problem, rather than relying on single 'big bang' interventions. Their cumulative impact appeared to be responsible for the progress that had been made so far. Second, problems were carefully targeted: for example, tackling crime by concentrating on specific crime types, or even specific burglars, as well as targeting small geographical areas and using situational measures to reduce opportunities and increase the likelihood of detection. Third, dedicated working groups to manage activity and regular meetings to review progress against targets were features of what had worked well. Fourth, partnership working was essential, both in the LSP and by services working together on the ground. However, partnership working was not unproblematic. To work well, the advantages of collaboration had to be clear, or it had to be a means of accessing additional funds. In education, the LSP was often perceived as not especially relevant given the policy focus on individual school performance, and for worklessness the LSP and especially neighbourhoods were seen as scales that needed to be complemented by a focus on the wider travel-to-work area. Sharing goals and funding were seen as ways of creating trust between partners, but there needed to be clarity about what needed to be done and by whom, and questions asked of those who were not meeting targets.

The teenage pregnancy floor target is a good example of the need for partnership working: in this case across the NHS, schools and employment services. In England, every top-tier local authority has a 10-year teenage pregnancy strategy jointly developed with the local NHS and other partners. Local work to reduce teenage conceptions and support teenage mothers is led by a teenage pregnancy coordinator working with a partnership board. In April 2001, extra resources to tackle the issue came with the Sure Start Plus initiative, launched in 35 targeted local authority areas as a five-year pilot to provide personalised advice and health services for pregnant teenagers and teenage parents (www.surestart.gov.uk).

Sure Start and Sure Start Plus are examples of a number of initiatives that focus on some of the same deprived areas as the NR strategy. Many programmes are now targeting young people in these areas, and there has been a growing recognition that they can be pursuing separate interventions among the same people. This is because risky behaviours tend to cluster together (Cohen et al, 2000). There therefore needs to be a youth policy that addresses the underlying causes of risky and antisocial behaviour among some young people. To a large extent this is seen by the government as a coordination issue (DfES, 2005). Improved coordination is certainly necessary but it needs to be user-led and properly resourced to be sufficient. More activities and services for young people are needed but in settings used by them. Furthermore, they should be accessible on a drop-in basis and, where appropriate, be provided in confidence.

Individual, personalised advice and support have been recognised as important in overcoming barriers to accessing services and jobs. This is an important strand of Sure Start Plus, for example, where specialist advisors work one to one with pregnant teenagers and teenage parents. A recent national evaluation found that the advisors were successful in addressing the crisis needs of pregnant and parenting young women, such as accommodation and emotional support, and in helping them to develop skills and prepare for parenting (Wiggins et al, 2005). Overall, however, the programme has proved less successful with achieving its stated objectives of reducing smoking and increasing breastfeeding, supporting participation in education, training or employment, and reaching and supporting fathers. The evaluators conclude that more time and resources would be needed to achieve these objectives. They also found a difference between local pilots that emphasised meeting targets and those that were needs led, taking their agenda from the young person themselves and their needs and circumstances. Pilots with a more target-led approach were more successful with achieving the programme's objective of raising educational achievement, although there was no evidence that this achieved a better long-term outcome. The health objectives were poorly met by all the pilots, regardless of their target-led or needs-led emphasis. The authors conclude that the factors behind this were more urgent needs to respond to crisis issues and the young people's emotional well-being, rather than raising issues about their health-related behaviours.

There is clearly a high risk of implementation deficit if targets do not make sense in the local practice context. But they are an essential aspect of any strategy to reduce inequality. Nottingham's LSP, for example, has formulated its teenage conceptions target as one of closing the gap between the fifth of wards with the highest under-18 conception rate and the average ward rate by at least 25% by 2010 (One City Partnership Nottingham, 2004). The city's teenage pregnancy rate is very high. The annual average number of conceptions to under-18-year-olds per 1,000 females aged 15-17 was 73.4 for 2001-03, compared to an average for all NR areas of 54.1, with its increasing trend in recent years going in the opposite direction to most other NR areas. Local analysis indicates that persistent non-attenders and young people excluded from school are particularly likely to become teenage parents, with an underlying issue of low aspirations and educational attainment. Out of school, they miss out on sex and relationship education (SRE) and access to support such as learning mentors, youth workers and school nursing.

Examples of interventions from Nottingham's 2004/05 strategy include a new chlamydia screening service operating in areas of highest need, combining screening with sexual health advice and family planning; a Healthy Schools programme focusing on teenage pregnancy and schools with the highest rates, training teachers to national SRE standards; and two community-based sexual health services run by the PCT and the local authority's Youth Service in areas with high teenage conception rates, with peer education schemes involving young people in delivering SRE alongside staff. In addition, Sure Start Plus is in contact with at least 50% of pregnant women under 18 and is aiming to increase this to 75% with NRF funding supporting the additional outreach activity.

This represents a significant effort to bring down Nottingham's teenage pregnancy rate. It is too early to say how successful this is being but clearly traditional sex education programmes in schools and other youth settings have not been successful in reducing high levels of teenage conceptions. There are two explanations for this: either agencies are not doing the right thing, or they are doing the right thing but not doing it right. Regarding the former, even well-delivered SRE will have little effect if a large part of the explanation for teenage conceptions among disadvantaged young women is that there are few concrete and hopeful alternatives. Young people need reasons for delaying intercourse and for the consistent use of contraception once they begin to have sex. Success therefore requires wide-ranging programmes linked into schools and neighbourhoods that can improve educational achievement and occupational opportunities and motivation. This is about establishing an environment that supports a future orientation, which was discussed in Chapter One, and implies further large-scale investment of resources in schools, colleges and jobs if teenage conception targets are to be met.

However, it is also likely that things have not been done right in Nottingham. A project in Brighton found that sex education programmes were often regarded as old-fashioned and irrelevant. They failed to recognise the role of drinking alcohol in risk-taking behaviour among young people who were generally sensible and well informed about unwanted pregnancies and sexually transmitted infections (Healthier Neighbourhoods Action Team, 2005). Local young people were supported in making a short film and resource pack that more realistically captured their experiences and could be shown in schools and other youth settings. Even so, cooperation from schools is needed for these initiatives, which can be difficult either because of other demands on teachers or resistance from governors. Reaching excluded young people and persistent non-attenders is a particular challenge.

A difficult task for NR and tackling health inequalities is to develop interventions based on evidence of what is likely to work. A first step is to target interventions where needs or risks are greatest, which means having a good knowledge of the local population. There has been impressive progress recently in the development of longitudinal and comparative data at a small-area level that can be used to monitor trends and differences in outcomes. Much of the data now available are for the fine-grained geography of Super Output Areas with their populations of around 1,500 people (www.ons.gov.uk). The usability of these data is improving with developments such as the 'Floor Targets Interactive' section of the NRU website (www.neighbourhoods.gov.uk) and data on clinical and health outcomes at www.nchod.nhs.uk. Very small areas can be picked out and targeted. However, it is important that these data are used knowledgeably. Life expectancy at birth, for example, is often used as an outcome measure but is an estimate that is subject to a margin of error. In small populations this can be wide, and a difference of two or three years between estimates of life expectancy for two areas may still not be statistically significant. Similarly, care must also be taken not to attach too much significance to changes over short time periods, especially if numbers are fairly small, so indicators such as teenage conceptions are normally calculated as three-year rolling averages. Other data such as benefit claims are counts that can be used to identify detailed geographies to map patterns of deprivation or ill-health (such as Incapacity Benefit claims) and target measures proactively, such as help with finding jobs.

There are still significant gaps in the data coverage of official statistics, such as health-related behaviours and mental health. Surveys can fill these but are costly and may not be effective for hard-to-reach groups and where there are problems of poor English literacy, suspicion about officialdom or difficulty making contact. Health data from primary care sources are likely to improve as part of the new Quality and Outcomes Framework, which collects a range of data associated with the performance management of new contracts for GP services (see www.ic.nhs.uk/services/qof) but data are not available for neighbourhoods. Without a survey it is currently impossible to measure important health indicators such as smoking prevalence at neighbourhood level. Smoking cessation services report data on quit rates but these say nothing about actual prevalence. An important objective of these services is to reduce premature deaths from cancer, but using cancer deaths as a measure means that any impact is unlikely to be demonstrable for some time, and would not be as direct a measure as the smoking rate. Synthetic estimates are sometimes used for health-related behaviours such as smoking, but these are not measures of actual outcomes. The timeliness of data is a further issue. This has been improving but teenage conceptions data, for instance, has a time lag of up to three years in availability from the Office of National Statistics. This means that for local monitoring purposes it is often still necessary to develop alternative sources, such as local NHS births data, which can be monitored on a virtually real-time basis.

Even with a strengthening capacity to make assessments of baselines and establish targets, there is still often a black box between what is being done on the ground and the outcome being aimed at, between actions and targets. Yet the large number of NR areas, and their common targets but different approaches, presents a natural laboratory for investigating what is working. For example, a commission for GO

North West that I recently undertook examined the performance of the region's 21 NRF LSPs with tackling health inequalities. There was a different pattern in performance across the LSPs for each of the three floor targets considered: premature deaths from circulatory diseases and cancers, and teenage conceptions. This pattern was not related to differences in the level of deprivation between the LSP areas. The variability in outcomes meant that QCA could be applied to looking for combinations of attributes associated with these outcomes. A survey was undertaken to gather data from the LSPs about their local contexts, their interventions and their ways of working. Respondents in each LSP assessed these features for the current time and for three years previously. The data for three years previously were used to take some account of the time lag in the availability of data for the health floor targets, so that the survey responses could be better compared with them. Data for the most recent five years were used to classify each LSP as to whether the relative gap in each floor target had recently been widening, staying much the same, or narrowing. Combinations of attributes were examined using fsQCA software and some clear patterns emerged.

The gap analysis for cancers compared under-75 mortality between each LSP and the non-NRF average for the North West over the period 1998-2000 to 2002-04 (these are three-year rolling averages). In ten of the 21 NRF LSPs the gap had been narrowing, in six it had been widening and in five it had been changing very little or not at all. These outcomes were compared with data from the survey, the population census and the MORI 'physical capital' index described in Chapter One, which is a score for the quality of the physical environment. Out of 35 variables, four distinguished the LSP areas where the gap had been narrowing from the other areas where the gap had been widening or staying much the same. One attribute, a high score on the physical capital index, was sufficient for the gap to have been narrowing. Either environmental quality or an unmeasured attribute associated with it appeared to create a receptive context for reducing cancer mortality. In other LSP areas where the gap had been narrowing but the physical capital score was lower, the attribute that these areas almost uniquely shared was that respondents assessed as good or exemplary their identification, understanding and targeting of inequalities. One LSP area where the gap had been narrowing shared neither the high physical capital nor the good/exemplary targeting attributes, but respondents assessed their joint working as about 'finding win–wins' *and* had proactive smoking cessation services working in the most deprived areas. This combination also applied to one other LSP area, but here the gap had *not* been narrowing. What was different about this LSP was that there was a major focus on acute care interventions. In none of the LSP areas without a high physical capital score, but where there was a major focus on acute care, had the gap been narrowing. This suggests that this attribute may describe a less effective focus in the locality on treatment rather than prevention.

Similar systematic patterns were evident for circulatory diseases and teenage conceptions, although with different combinations of context and ways of working making a difference. For example, three attributes were associated with narrowing the teenage conceptions gap. An absence of high population turnover was necessary but not sufficient. All LSP areas where the gap had been narrowing combined an absence of high population turnover with teenage conceptions being a high priority and a major emphasis on lifestyle interventions. The method is exploratory but illustrates the potential of QCA for evaluating performance in a way that considers possible causal combinations of contextual, policy and practice attributes. This has the potential to provide a basis for the exchange of good practice and an understanding of the contextual issues that programmes face. In the North West, there were also encouraging results about change over the three-year period that respondents considered when making their assessments. The attributes that were associated with better performance were appreciably more common at the time the survey was completed (March 2006) than three years previously.

Whether an intervention works can either be investigated as rigorously as possible or approached on a 'good-enough' basis. Frequently limited resources mean that the latter is the only feasible option. As discussed further in Chapter Seven, the 'theory of change' approach can be used with data that may not be the most desirable methodologically but can be expected to track relevant change. Thus, we can identify indicators to track outcomes, such as the gap in premature CHD deaths between the worst 20% of neighbourhoods and the city average; indicators to track the drivers of these outcomes, such as diet, smoking and physical activity if these can be obtained from survey data; indicators to describe the context of intervention, such as the level of deprivation or BME representation in the population from the IMD and census; and descriptions of the interventions and how they are delivered, such as a physical activity programme delivered in target neighbourhoods or among an 'at-risk' group, or screening and early treatment programmes with or without active outreach and inreach work. We can then compare these data with a theory of how we expect them to relate causally: what combination of drivers, contexts, programmes and ways of delivering programmes are associated with what outcomes? This is, in other words, Ragin's (2000) method of QCA. It also allows for combinations of interventions to be considered, which is how in reality interventions are normally delivered.

Local governance in conditions of causal complexity

LSPs are intended to be central to local governance in England. They have an expanding role as 'the partnership of partnerships', preparing Community Strategies as the overarching local plan for their areas, and being expected to deliver LAAs as the Community Strategy's action plan (ODPM, 2005e). In the NRF areas, LSPs are pivotal in the local implementation of the national NR strategy.

LSPs have been established in each of England's local authority areas to improve public services and establish a framework of shared accountability for service improvements and outcomes. They are voluntary associations across most of the country but are required in NRF areas, where they are expected to prioritise the most disadvantaged neighbourhoods and groups with action plans based on the national floor targets and other local targets that they may adopt, supported by NRF allocations. LSPs currently have no statutory powers and rely on those of their partner agencies. They are generally led by the local authority in partnership with other agencies such as the local NHS PCT, the police, the employment service and community, voluntary sector and business representatives. LSPs are vehicles for elected local authorities to exercise their community leadership role. This is expected to be done 'in partnership rather than by command' (ODPM, 2005e, p 10). Particular emphasis is placed by the government on the role of LSPs as a means of involving local residents and businesses in governance, and achieving coordination across the several separate partnerships that exist in areas such as crime reduction and children's and youth services, as well as any NDC or Neighbourhood Management partnership in their area. They operate through a number of theme or working groups, which is likely to include a health partnership.

LSPs are expected to be inclusive bodies representing all the key stakeholders in a local authority area, with the work of their boards informed by that of the thematic and neighbourhood partnerships and managed through a smaller executive board. The LSP's aims, priorities and targets are brought together in a Community Strategy, which must be consulted upon locally. In theory, and to a growing extent in practice, the Community Strategy should provide a framework through which partner organisations can assist each other in meeting their own targets as well as shared cross-cutting targets. Specific commitments are formalised as Local Public Service Agreements (LPSAs) reached between the local partners and the government, underpinning the Treasury's insistence that increased public expenditure is conditional on setting targets that enable progress to be measured and evaluated. LPSAs, in fact, include a financial incentive in that the local authority receives a 'reward grant' if it achieves the agreed performance improvement beyond that expected without the LPSA, and this can be shared with a partner agency such as a PCT.

There are, however, concerns about LSPs, ranging from the quality of their leadership and their capacity to get things done to their accountability. The latter includes issues about weak cultures of performance management and deficiencies in how well LSPs consult local people, who only have the opportunity to elect one of the partners, the local authority. Despite this, the role of LSPs is evolving quickly, and the government in England sees their new responsibilities as part of the solution to their weaknesses. There are two particularly significant developments in this respect. The first is the evolution of Community Strategies to *Sustainable* Community Strategies and their action plans, LAAs. The second is the development of inspection, the reviewing and assessing of local public services.

Both of these represent a consolidation of local governance as about partnership working. This is conducted within an overarching and increasingly area- and outcome-based performance management framework, contrasting with an earlier services- and processes-based model. England is currently taking a different course in this respect compared to the other countries of the UK where inspection is less developed, but partnership working is a common theme and expectation.

The new title for Community Strategies signifies that they 'take a more cross-disciplinary and integrated approach to social, economic and environmental issues', with a clear process of 'baselining current performance', using evidence and forecasting (ODPM, 2005e, pp 17-18). Following a recent review of policy approaches to deprived areas, there is a heightened expectation that in the NR areas the Sustainable Community Strategy will be a plan for sustainable development (Cabinet Office, 2005). This means bringing a cross-agency focus to bear on three areas in particular: jobs, encouraging enterprise and private sector investment; improving public services and outcomes; and avoiding 'clustering poor people in poor places', creating more mixed-income communities. These priorities follow from an analysis that highlighted how weak local economies drive area deprivation, failures in how well local services meet the needs of disadvantaged residents, and the role of housing allocation systems and town planning in both creating and breaking up concentrations of deprivation. The review's analysis of concentrations of deprivation argues that it is more difficult for people living in these areas to utilise the personal contacts that are an important route into employment, for children to do well at school without the benefit of more mixed school intakes, and to tackle drug use and crime when these are more likely to spread and be 'peer induced'.

The Sustainable Community Strategy sets out the strategic vision and priorities for the area, while LAAs set out the detailed outcomes, indicators and targets that relate to the strategy and how its delivery will be funded (ODPM, 2005e). Local authorities, working through their LSPs, agree the LAA with national government, with the LAA usually organised into four blocks. These are children and young people, safer and stronger communities, healthier communities and older people, and economic development and enterprise. Increasingly the LSP's sub-partnerships are being aligned with these blocks, and it seems likely that there will be further budget flexibility between them. The idea is to create less 'budget silos', rationalise indicators and targets, and encourage collaboration and innovation, including shared priorities such as health inequalities. LAAs are being rolled out nationally in England following a pilot phase, which has been evaluated favourably overall. The pilot led to 'better dialogue and joint planning in areas requiring partnership action, such as public health and community safety.... The process strengthened partnership working locally and helped partners to resolve issues where they had previously been unable to agree' (Office of Public Management et al, 2005, p 105).

Plsek (2001) defines the features of complex organisational systems in terms of adaptability within the boundaries of a few rules locally applied, working with a 'good-enough' vision that leaves space for innovation and experimentation in meeting the system's goals. Feedback – from performance indicators and evaluations – is necessary to track whether progress is being made in the right direction. Partnerships are complex systems and the development of this mode of governance is to be expected in increasingly complex societies. Policy making is adapting to the world in which it is now operating (Chapman, 2004). It is not surprising that partnership working has developed as a way of recognising that the transformational capacity of any single agency in tackling wicked issues such as health inequalities needs to operate through networks and 'governed interdependence'. Weiss (2003) observes that this is a feature of contemporary 'risk societies', where complexity outstrips the capacity of single agencies of government to act on their own.

LSPs are meant to reach out to the private sector and to voluntary and community groups, bringing them round the table on an equal footing with statutory agencies. Local people are recognised in the policy documents as part of any solution but sharing power with community groups can be problematic, despite the availability of dedicated resources to support community involvement in NRF LSPs. It could, however, become more problematic with LAAs because there is a growing local authority view that they need smaller boards comprised only of the major spending agencies locally. This accountability issue has recently been rising up the policy agenda.

The present government's solution to the accountability issue is the second significant development to affect LSPs after Sustainable Community Strategies and LAAs. The solution is the 'joining up' of inspection and an enhanced role for 'local pressure' to drive service improvement, with somewhat less emphasis on national targets and accountability (ODPM, 2005e). Inspection has expanded in the public sector as a means of demonstrating to government and the public that services are performing well and improving. Local authorities are responsible for the delivery of Community Strategies, LAAs and local NR strategies, but must work through their LSPs. However, both local authorities and their major partner agencies such as PCTs have their own inspection regimes. In addition, NRF LSPs are required to have a Performance Management Framework in place that keeps under review both outcomes and partnership working, together with an improvement plan. These frameworks are extending to LAAs to bring shared accountability. The current government view is that:

> It is integral to our vision for the long-term future of LSPs, and local governance more generally, that the space for individual local agencies to act innovatively and collaboratively is increased through a reduction in the level of organisation-based/national targets. The method of working is being facilitated by the area-based approach to performance management introduced by the LAA and a similar approach in specific areas, for example, children's trusts are moving to an area-based approach to performance management. This is underpinned by cross-agency working

with a duty to improve children's well being. (ODPM, 2005e, p 38)

Children's trusts are meant to bring together the education, health and social services for children and young people in an area as a 'whole system', with multidisciplinary teams and co-location in settings such as children's centres and extended schools. This reform has been driven by viewing services from the perspective of the young user, emphasising integration and responsiveness. It has also driven a recasting of inspection, with new Joint Area Reviews (JARs) replacing the separate inspections of local education authorities, social services and Connexions services for young people. This adaptation of audit to areas as well as organisations is also likely to extend to cross-cutting public health topics such as accidents, with in this case the Healthcare Commission and Audit Commission working jointly to review performance in a local area.

The user perspective is an important driver for integration and is at the centre of Jake Chapman's critique of public sector 'system failure' (Chapman, 2004). Chapman applies complexity theory to his analysis of the failures of mechanistic and reductionist thinking in public policy, which in his view has created a burdensome administrative load without securing significant improvements. His main criticism is of targets:

> Target-setting may be a short-term way to stimulate and focus efforts to improve performance. However, a specific target can encapsulate only one element of a complex organisation, and its dominance is likely to undermine other aspects of the organisation that are crucial to its general and long-term effectiveness. An example is the apparent link between the ambitious performance targets and heavy measurement in schools policy and the continuous difficulties faced by the school system in motivating and retaining qualified teachers. (Chapman, 2004, p 58)

Public policy issues are often complex, and this creates situations where mechanistic cause–effect thinking does not work, often because of unanticipated feedbacks. Another of Chapman's examples is police action to stem the supply of drugs: feedback can force up prices and encourage cutting the drugs with other substances, exacerbating crime to pay for the higher prices and health risks from the cut drugs. These unintended consequences undermine the original intervention. There are plenty of other examples: one reported at the time of writing is the unexpectedly high cost of incentive payments to GPs to meet targets, including prevention and public health targets such as providing smoking cessation advice. These targets appear to have been rather too easy, leading to GPs 'overachieving' and paradoxically squeezing NHS budgets for major programmes of screening and other public health initiatives (Timmins, 2005).

Of course, this last example is also one of where targets have worked – GPs are doing more early treatment, rehabilitation and preventative work, and are now strongly incentivised with cash payments to do this. Targets in general seem to have worked in bringing down waiting times for NHS treatment (see Chapter Six) and can be reviewed, made tougher or further incentivised if necessary. A key issue, however, is whether the right things are being done. GPs are now paid for giving their patients smoking cessation advice, with targets for increasing (often very sharply) the number of smokers who quit after receiving a smoking cessation service. However, as discussed in Chapter Two, these services appear to have relatively little to offer in reducing smoking prevalence, especially socioeconomic inequalities in smoking, despite their cost-effectiveness. For Chapman it is necessary to consider overall system performance. In relation to smoking that means focusing on smoking bans and improving working and living conditions, with a supporting role for cessation services.

System improvement for Chapman means actively engaging service providers with continuously improving the system based on learning from end-user feedback. This means not treating providers in instrumental ways, rewarded or punished according to the results of performance assessments. Echoing the results of the floor targets evaluation discussed above (GFA Consulting, 2005), Chapman argues that the evidence points to change coming from stakeholders' continuous engagement with sustainable improvement over a long period, making incremental progress. This typically involves trying multiple approaches and letting direction come out of gradually shifting attention towards those things that seem to be working best.

While this notion of incremental change appears to conflict with the emphasis in complexity theory on change occurring as non-linear transitions in quality, this is partly a question of timeframe. Over time, a transformation may indeed be evident. This can come from small changes: while complexity theory suggests that change in key parameters is what brings a system to a tipping point, parameter change can be an emergent outcome of many changes at a lower level. If these changes align with an overall goal, their total effect may well be what is known in complexity thinking as fractal emergence. While most emergence is context and interaction driven, with uncertain outcomes, fractal emergence has more alignment between local actions and the emergent outcome. This is a result of many purposeful actions moving the system towards a common goal. Fractal emergence is ultimately the aim of programmes that have many local variations but are oriented to a few key outcomes.

The direction of travel in the reform of inspection is consistent with Chapman's analysis, and there is little doubt that this type of thinking is having an influence on policy. The introduction of Comprehensive Performance Assessment (CPA) in 2002 as the inspection regime for local government was a shift away from 'silos' to assessing the overall performance and capacity of the local authority as a single system, an approach since extended to the new Children's Services Joint *Area* Reviews (ODPM, 2005e; emphasis added). According to a recent consultation paper on inspection, there is 'growing recognition in inspection methodologies of the responsibilities of organisations to work in partnership better, to secure the joined-up outcomes which users expect' (ODPM, 2005e, p 11). Thus, inspections of local authorities will assess the quality of their partnership working through CPA, with PCTs similarly assessed through the Healthcare Commission.

While cross-cutting targets raise an issue about who is accountable for making progress with them, in practice these targets are usually owned by a lead agency. Health is an example, with the local PCT generally leading on the health targets for an area. The wider determinants of health, however, are upstream from the health care interventions with which PCTs are primarily concerned, given their main role in commissioning health care services. PCTs do not commission housing services, for example, which are likely to have a more upstream contribution to make to tackling health inequalities. Therefore, health and housing services need to have health inequalities as a shared priority. Some service-specific objectives that the housing service has will support the PCT's objectives, and vice versa; in other words, cause–effect relationships extend across service boundaries. This is the 'golden thread' of shared performance management. A housing organisation's programme of work to meet the decent homes standard, for example, will include several objectives and actions relevant to health, from installing new kitchens, which is an opportunity to intervene with healthy eating initiatives, to double glazing and insulation, and their potential to reduce cold-related morbidity. By mapping these linkages between organisations certain objectives and actions will stand out as important to the performance of more than one organisation, enabling these to be prioritised for monitoring and (shared) resourcing. This approach is already informing the design of performance management systems, such as InPhase's *PerformancePlus™* (www.inphase.com/performanceplus.htm).

England's strategy for tackling health inequalities is set out in *Tackling Health Inequalities: A Programme for Action*, recently built on by the *Choosing Health* White Paper and supported by *Tackling Health Inequalities: What Works*, which identifies effective interventions for health priority areas (DH, 2003, 2004a, 2005c). As noted in Chapter One, there is an emphasis on providing more opportunities, support and information for people to make 'healthy choices'. The NR strategy is a recognition that these choices are affected by the physical, cultural and commercial environments in which people live, and that partnership working which tackles issues together, rather than in isolation, is needed (SEU, 2001, p 5). As well as recognising inequality, and adopting measurable targets to narrow inequality across a range of fronts, the NR strategy aims to change local governance. This is as ambitious, if not more so, than the outcomes defined by the floor targets. The aim is that the most deprived areas see faster improvements in outcomes than the rest of the country, but in the process local systems of policy making and service delivery are expected to change significantly.

These changes in governance include much more attention to data and tracking change. As part of a programme of substantially improving the availability of small-area statistics, the NRU maintains a web-based system called Floor Targets Interactive that enables progress towards the PSA floor targets to be monitored (www.neighbourhoods.gov.uk). The system covers all English local authorities down to district level, but the focus is on the local authorities that receive support from the NRF. There is a large amount of overlap between these areas and the areas of the country with the worst health and deprivation indicators included in the Spearhead Group of areas by the Department of Health, with a similar aim of closing the gap with the rest of the country. It is this infrastructure for identifying, targeting and monitoring geographical inequality beyond a few designated areas that makes these measures different from past social and urban policies in the UK.

Is this working? The broad picture is one of some progress at this stage, as already reviewed above. Other evidence is available from the NDC programme, which began earlier than the NR strategy in 1998. The NDC programme targets 39 of the most deprived neighbourhoods in England, with populations of around 10,000 people and budgets over 10 years of about £50 million each. Results from national evaluators are available, including survey data (CRESR, 2005). They conclude that community engagement has been much better than past ABIs because it has received significant attention, including with BME groups. The statistical indicators, however, show fairly modest change. Across the NDC areas, fear of burglary fell from 65% in 2002 to 55% in 2004. The proportion of residents reporting that they were satisfied with their area rose from 60% to 66%. Fourteen per cent more respondents in 2004 compared to 2002 reported that the area had improved in the past two years. Forty-five per cent of residents who said in 2002 that they would move had changed their minds by 2004. Rates of people moving off unemployment and sickness benefits were higher than rates for the rest of the country.

The picture is less good for health outcomes. In 2002, only 43% of residents reported their health as good, 16% less than the national average. It is ambitious to expect any significant change in morbidity and especially mortality over such a short period of time as health interventions can take many years to show effects. Indeed, no improvement is yet evident in the NDC areas. Of more concern is that the NDC surveys enable health-related behaviours to be tracked and there is little or no evidence of lifestyle change, for example in smoking or exercise. Satisfaction with health care services increased by a few percentage points but was already quite high. There are four key outcomes for the NDC programme: housing and the physical environment; employment, income and enterprise; crime and disorder; and health. Of these, health is where change is not much in evidence so far .

At present, the only health outputs audited for the NDC programme are 'number of people benefiting from healthy lifestyle projects', 'number of people benefiting from new or improved health facilities', and 'number of new or improved health facilities'. These indicators are of little value in determining either the contribution of local health services to the objective of narrowing the health inequalities gap between the NDC areas and the country as a whole, or the health gain from wider measures such as housing improvements. For housing, the audited outputs are 'number of homes improved or built' and 'number of traffic calming schemes'. These are potentially important public health measures but we need to know whether they are working to reduce health inequalities.

This is not just an issue for the renewal of existing neighbourhoods but for new neighbourhoods as well. Chapter Four discussed the neighbourhood concept informing the major expansion of new housing at North Harlow. As part of the landowner's strategy for developing the land as an exemplary sustainable development, a series of principles have been developed for the new community's health services based on stakeholder and expert consultation (www.harlownorth.com). These include integrating design targets for access to green space, amenities and public transport into neighbourhood, master and delivery plans; adopting the Lifetime Homes Standard where possible; equitable access to health care within 5-10 minutes by foot or public transport, with local participation in shaping services; and the use of health and well-being indicators. There is also an intention to join up health services with wider agendas, such as the local hospital procuring food locally to assist with regenerating agricultural communities and reducing food miles, and cutting waste.

Conclusion: evaluation lessons

The proposed development of Harlow North is informed by evidence about what is likely to work best for people's health. Beyond health care provision, this is still frequently not thought through when renewing deprived neighbourhoods, despite the evidence that was reviewed in Chapter Four. It is, however, difficult to attribute cause when investigating the effects of neighbourhood renewal. For example, progress with reducing teenage conceptions may depend less on dedicated services than the success of mainstream reform of what is taught in schools, and the aspirations for higher education or employment instilled in young people who may otherwise become disengaged and leave education early. The difficulties involved with evaluating complex interventions are discussed by Barnes, M. et al (2005) in their account of the national evaluation of HAZs, one of the first significant ABIs launched by the New Labour government in 1998. This chapter concludes with the HAZ story because it brings together some of the key points in the chapter about targets and interventions, and how it is not only necessary to be explicit about both, but also about the causal processes believed to link them.

HAZs covered large populations; the smallest was Luton with a population of 200,000 and the largest was Merseyside with 1.4 million people. They were funded to tackle health inequality by promoting change in how services operated, especially building collaboration across organisations and with the public. Complexity arose from the organisational structures in the HAZ localities, the ways in which issues manifested themselves, how solutions were framed, and how policies were developed locally and nationally. The evaluation needed to recognise HAZs as a national initiative implemented in local contexts. These contexts each had different histories and circumstances, and these would affect HAZ implementation over time. Features of the local context that made an appreciable difference to outcomes were the existence of substantial minority ethnic communities, lack of coterminosity across organisational boundaries, competition between agencies, high turnovers of key staff, and the role of key personalities as either champions or blockers (Benzeval, 2005).

When the processes of implementation were studied it was clear that change did not occur in a linear sequence but through continuous processes of interaction and adjustment to changing circumstances. The many agents involved in HAZ work made attributing 'who did what and when to what effect' extremely difficult. Yet this 'kaleidoscope of local activity' was a strength of the initiative (Judge and Bauld, 2005, p 189). Process outcomes were important, and certainly more feasible over the lifetime of the HAZs than making significant measurable progress with closing gaps in health inequalities. HAZs had their greatest success in getting equity issues onto the agendas of a wide range of agencies, but little strategic change occurred as a result, and other 'must dos' often received greater priority. There is no robust evidence that HAZs achieved greater improvements to population health than other comparable areas. A lack of baseline data, and of any targets that could realistically be tackled by local interventions, meant that the apparent ineffectiveness of HAZs appeared to be a planning failure.

The HAZ initiative suffered from a lack of consistent purpose nationally and planning weaknesses locally. This made evaluation difficult. Nationally, following the arrival of a new Secretary of State for Health, HAZs were expected to swing behind meeting national targets for reducing heart disease and cancer, despite an original brief to focus on local priorities (Bauld et al, 2005). Locally, the first national evaluation report commented, 'Only in very rare cases is it possible to identify a clear and logical pathway which links problems, strategies for intervention, milestones or targets with associated time-scales and longer-term outcomes ... specific "targets" were highlighted without any accompanying explanation of the mechanisms intended to achieve them' (Judge et al, 1999, pp 30-1). Putting this right for future interventions would not only make evaluation easier but strengthen the prospect of success because thinking has been done to identify plausible change pathways that can then be monitored.

Following cuts in their budgets the role of HAZs was eroded. This was eventually terminal with the launch of the NR strategy as England's overarching framework for local partnership working to tackle area deprivation, as well as major restructuring of the NHS itself. The latter saw HAZ projects absorbed into the newly created local PCTs. The evaluation certainly casts light on issues of organisation: organisational configurations, organisational leadership, organisational capacity and organisational change. These were all in Stacey's (2003) zone of complexity, where there is a lack of certainty or agreement about outcomes and how inputs are causally related to them. HAZs had a 'whole-system' approach to the areas in which they were based, in which different ways of working as much as extra resources were the policy inputs. The main lessons learned in terms of local intervention were the lack of clarity and consistency about objectives, the lack of clarity about how outcomes would be achieved, and the overly short timescales in which health improvements were expected. Overall, however, Bauld et al (2005) cast doubt on the ability of any relatively short-term programmatic approach to deliver change in a complex 'wicked issue' like health inequalities. They argue instead for a dedicated national policy focus on health inequalities, and it is to this issue that we turn in the next chapter.

SIX

Health inequality as a policy priority

The Black report, published in 1980, is often cited as the key reference point for when health inequality was placed on the national policy agenda in the UK (Black et al, 1980). Its recommendations, however, were rejected as too costly by the then Conservative government which the previous year had replaced the Labour administration that had commissioned the report. Health inequality, though, would not go away as an issue, with continuing pressure from public health movements such as the WHO's 'Health for All' campaign and Healthy Cities Project (Ashton and Seymour, 1988). Nevertheless, public health policy under the Conservatives concentrated on specific disease prevention strategies rather than health inequalities or the wider determinants of health beyond individual lifestyles. Targets for reducing both major diseases and individual risk factors were set out in England's *Health of the Nation* strategy (DH, 1992). The strategy acknowledged 'health variations' that were linked to socioeconomic factors but essentially dismissed the issue as not well understood.

Labour returned to power in 1997 and, in social policy, developed alongside a number of new national measures a swathe of ABIs aimed at tackling 'social exclusion', including the NR strategy and HAZs (SEU, 2001; Barnes, M. et al, 2005). The new government commissioned an update of the evidence on health inequality from a working group led by Professor Donald Acheson, which reported in 1998 (Acheson, 1998). This recommended evaluating all public policies for their impact on health inequalities, prioritising the health of families with children because of the significance of early-life influences on health, and taking further measures to tackle health inequalities and improve the living standards of poorer households. The report was followed by a new national strategy for England, *Saving Lives: Our Healthier Nation* (Secretary of State for Health, 1998) and in Scotland and Wales, which from 1998 had devolved governments with responsibility for health policy, by *Towards a Healthier Scotland* (Secretary of State for Scotland, 1999) and *Better Health: Better Wales* (Secretary of State for Wales, 1998). Targets were set in these strategies for reducing death rates from cancer, CHD and stroke, accidents and mental illness.

The strategies also recognised the importance of tackling social, economic and environmental factors, and of partnership working between the NHS, local government and the voluntary and community sectors.

In England, a national policy focus on health inequalities arrived for the NHS with *The NHS Plan* (DH, 2000b). The Plan clearly recognised health inequalities as an issue right across the NHS, as well as the need to work in partnership with other public services to reduce them. National health inequality targets were announced in 2001 and *Tackling Health Inequalities: A Programme for Action* (DH, 2003) followed in July 2003. The centrepiece of this strategy was clear objectives to reduce socioeconomic and geographical inequalities in infant mortality and life expectancy, incorporated as PSA targets to be reached by 2010. The strategy sets out four key themes of supporting families, mothers and children; engaging communities and individuals in improving health; prevention and providing effective treatment and care; and tackling the underlying determinants of poor health. Partnership working is again emphasised, especially at the local level through the work of LSPs.

Further impetus was given to the effort to reduce health inequalities by reports commissioned by the Treasury from Derek Wanless, ex-Chief Executive of National Westminster Bank, on the long-term funding requirements of the NHS (Wanless, 2002, 2004). Wanless concluded that funding for the NHS needed to continue to expand in real terms, but also that the public needed to be 'fully engaged' with prevention to help contain rising demands for health care. In particular, Wanless identified the importance of making progress with improving the health of the most disadvantaged groups in the population, with the worst health status.

A shift in emphasis occurred with the publication in 2004 of the government's public health White Paper, *Choosing Health* (DH, 2004a). This created more distance between approaches in England and those of the new Scottish and Welsh governments. The emphasis on reducing health inequality is still very much in place, but the White Paper is imbued with a wider agenda of enabling people to exercise choice, rather than have choices made for them by regulation or 'one size fits all' public services. In large measure this reflects the political strategy of New Labour in aiming to head off attacks from the Conservative opposition by recasting the welfare state not as a welfare bureaucracy but as personalised services offering choice. The competition that choice generates is also seen as a way of driving service improvements. This political factor is absent in Scotland and Wales, where the dominance of left-of-centre and nationalist politics and the absence of any major Conservative vote have meant that market-based approaches have so far been largely eschewed in favour of local planning and partnerships.

Choosing Health argues that people want governments to support them in making choices that are good for their health rather than have these choices made for them. It attempts to strike a balance between choice, not allowing choice to harm or inconvenience others, and targeting services so that they help disadvantaged groups make healthy choices and access the services they need. Specific measures include personal health trainers to reach people who find a change in health-related lifestyle most difficult, a ban on smoking in enclosed public spaces, but with exemptions for pubs not serving food and private clubs where people can choose to go and smoke, and designation of the Spearhead Group of PCTs in the 70 local authority areas with the worst population health. Exempting clubs and pubs not serving food from the smoking ban attracted considerable criticism, not least because a disproportionate number are located in deprived areas. When this came before Parliament in March 2006 the partial ban was extended to a full smoking ban in enclosed public spaces and workplaces against a background of strong lobbying by public health groups.

Choosing Health is backed by PSA targets, and over half of the new targets are about health improvement rather than treatment. Some are joint targets: reducing childhood obesity is shared between the Departments of Health, for Education and Skills, and for Culture, Media and Sport, and cutting teenage conceptions is shared between the Departments of Health and for Education and Skills. A delivery plan, published in March 2005, again emphasises health improvement as a shared priority right across the public services (DH, 2005d). PCTs are expected to include in their Local Delivery Plans (LDPs) actions to reduce smoking and alcohol dependency, improve levels of physical activity and reduce obesity, modernise sexual health services, introduce health trainers, and develop the NHS workforce. Much of the delivery is expected to be in partnership with local authorities and other partners, with LAAs formalising this. Several shared priorities are identified by *Choosing Health* where neighbourhood renewal can contribute to health improvement by promoting walking, play and mental health in 'cleaner, safer, greener communities' and improving access to services. In NRF areas, LAAs must include outcomes and indicators that relate to the six NR strategy themes of crime, education, housing, worklessness, liveability and health. The health outcome is: 'Reduce premature mortality rates, and reduce inequalities in premature mortality rates between wards/neighbourhoods, with a particular focus on reducing the risk factors for heart disease, stroke, and related diseases (CVD) (smoking, diet and physical activity)' (NRU Health Team, 2006, p 1).

The role of performance management

Of particular significance in New Labour's health inequalities policy is that delivery is performance managed. Performance management based on targets and inspection has evolved rapidly in recent years in the UK. The Audit Commission was set up in 1982 with the remit of keeping the economy and efficiency of local government services in England under review, and its focus shifted from a preoccupation with efficiency in the 1980s to a concern with effectiveness in the 1990s (Blackman, 1995). This was reflected in the Commission's first list of performance indicators that local authorities have had to collect and publish annually since 1993/94. In 1990, the Audit Commission's role was extended to include NHS organisations and, in 1992, targets were introduced by the then Conservative government's *Health of the Nation* strategy for disease prevention and health promotion. These were targets for improvements in five priority areas against which local health authorities were expected to perform: circulatory diseases, cancers, mental health, HIV/AIDS and accidents (DH, 1992).

Along with the development of policy since 1997, from first recognising health inequalities as a policy priority to then formulating targets for narrowing inequalities, has been the expansion of performance management into health inequalities (Acheson, 1998; DH, 1998, 2003, 2004b). Performance management in the NHS and local government has led to a sharper focus on priorities and to improved performance where targets apply (Audit Commission, 2003; Crisp, 2003). The Healthcare Commission, in its 2005 annual report on the state of health care in England, concluded that many measurable improvements to health care could be attributed to targets (Healthcare Commission, 2005a). Some services that had not performed so well, including mental health, sexual health, and maternity and dental services, were where there was a lack of targets or requirements to collect information. This assessment is largely supported in an analysis by Bevan and Hood (2006), who found that the strong performance management of waiting-time targets in England appeared to have meant better improvements than in the lighter audit regimes of Scotland and Wales. Those improvements that have occurred in the latter two countries appear partly to have been influenced by indirect pressure from the policy of naming and shaming in England.

Whether targets and their performance management can extend successfully to wicked issues like health inequalities, however, is still an open question. The difficulty of measuring all the dimensions of the quality of a service is magnified considerably for a wicked issue that cuts across services. Yet the principle of 'management by objectives' first expounded by Drucker (1954) seems transferable if an outcome can be defined. Indeed, in 1984 the WHO European Region secured governmental endorsement for 38 'Health for All' targets, and a number of governments followed with their own national targets for health improvement. The development of targets as policy tools to focus programmes on health improvement objectives reflected advances in public health research demonstrating relationships between risk factors and health outcomes. It followed that it should be possible to set targets and expect programmes to be put in place to meet them within defined timeframes. Improvements in the availability of data and in data technologies also enabled much better monitoring and assessment of performance, so that baselines and milestones could be defined quantitatively.

While performance assessment is the process of monitoring and reviewing progress against targets, performance management uses progress against targets as a basis for intervention, often in the form of either rewards or sanctions. The UK, Australia, New Zealand and Canada have been early leaders in the public sector, followed by other countries seeking to achieve improvements in the performance of their public services, from Japan to China (Wye, 2002). Globalisation has fuelled this trend, with greater pressure on public services to demonstrate outcomes for the public funds they receive, and the global development of information and communication technology that can support performance-based management systems and the spread of ideas and practices. Few managers of public services are now without responsibility for a set of targets that they are held accountable for achieving.

The positive impacts of this audit culture include encouraging improvement, greater accountability to the public and politicians, diagnosing success and failure, providing lessons for others, and discouraging wrong or ineffective actions because of the prospect of external scrutiny (Davis et al, 2001). The negative effects, however, include the costs of complying with audit, the crowding out of innovation and creativity as too risky, damage to staff morale, and the distraction from basic service delivery. Performance indicators can also have dysfunctional effects, notably gaming (Smith, 1995; Public Administration Select Committee, 2003; Bird et al, 2005). Managers may focus on performance at the borderline of a performance threshold, or give priority to narrow areas of performance that are likely to impact on the performance measures but have negative consequences for other aspects of the service. Reported performance improves but there is little or no real improvement. Performance data have also been criticised for a lack of robustness and systematic auditing (Bevan and Hood, 2006).

Amid these academic, professional and political criticisms of performance management, New Labour has sought to adapt its approach while not losing the basic principle of transparent accountability for implementing policy objectives down the delivery chain (Public Administration Select Committee, 2003). There is a constant tension in this respect between nationally-set objectives and locally determined priorities. In the NHS, a new Priorities and Planning Framework (PPF) published by the Department of Health in July 2004 as *National Standards, Local Action* marked a shift away from a large number of national targets towards giving greater scope for local priority and target setting (DH, 2004b). The intention was to encourage local flexibility and innovation within a more rationalised framework of uniform standards of quality for NHS services across the country. However, following the 2004 Spending Review the health inequality targets were expanded. The targets for life expectancy and infant mortality were retained and new floor targets were added for cancer, CVD and smoking reduction. A new target for halting the rise in obesity among children under 11 was also introduced. These considerably strengthened the Department of Health's PSA to tackle health inequalities. If there is a strategy behind these shifts in the number of targets in England, it is that there is an easing off regarding the number of targets for health care, as performance has improved, but an expansion of targets for health inequalities, where performance is a much more recently recognised issue (especially local variations in closing gaps) and still a problem.

The PSA targets for health inequalities are complemented by 12 'national headline indicators' selected to monitor progress at national and local levels with tackling the underlying drivers of preventable mortality (see Table 6.1). Some of these have an explicit connection to policy programmes, such as the housing and child poverty indicators, while for others the causal connections are more complex, such as deaths rates from circulatory disease.

The PPF is not prescriptive regarding the local approaches taken to

Table 6.1: National headline indicators for health inequalities, England

Issue	Indicator
Access to primary care	Number of primary care professionals per 100,000 population
Accidents	Road accident casualty rates in disadvantaged communities
Child poverty	Proportion of children living in low-income households
Diet	Proportion of people consuming five or more portions of fruit and vegetables per day in the lowest quintile of household income distribution
Education	Proportion of those aged 16 achieving qualifications equivalent to 5 GCSEs at grades A* to C
Homelessness	Number of homeless families with children living in temporary accommodation
Housing	Proportion of households living in non-decent housing (a government housing standard)
Influenza vaccinations	Percentage uptake of flu vaccinations by older people (aged 65 plus)
PE and school sport	Percentage of school children who spend a minimum of two hours each week on high quality PE and school sport within and beyond the curriculum
Smoking prevalence	Prevalence of smoking among people in manual social groups and among pregnant women
Teenage conceptions	Rate of under-18 conceptions
Mortality from the major killer diseases	Age-standardised death rates per 100,000 population aged under 75 for cancer and circulatory diseases (for the 20% of areas with the highest rates compared to the national average)

Source: Department of Health (2005c)

address the national priorities, beyond requiring action to accord with key principles such as partnership working and targeting. PCTs are also expected to agree additional targets, based on local priorities, with local authorities and other partners through the LSP, creating the linkage with NR programmes. The PPF does define a set of national standards that NHS organisations are assessed against, organised in seven 'domains', the seventh of which is public health. While there are aspects relevant to reducing health inequalities across all the domains, there is a particular focus on reducing health inequalities in the seventh domain. The standards are also divided between 'core standards', which represent current expectations about what is delivered, and 'developmental standards', which are targets for improvement. The latter are regarded as important as measures of improving quality as the government pursues its strategy of making considerable additional investment in the NHS up to 2008 (after which it is widely expected that funding increases will be more modest).

The Healthcare Commission was launched in April 2004 with a wide-ranging mandate to assess the quality and value for money of health services, and to promote improvements. Its prime focus is on the core and developmental standards. It conducts reviews called 'annual health checks' of all NHS organisations, considering both core and developmental standards, as well as undertaking 'improvement reviews' by theme or geographical area. The annual health checks result in published ratings for each local NHS trust. Each PCT makes a self-assessment of whether it believes it is in compliance with each core standard, which is then evaluated by the Healthcare Commission with reference to a wide range of mostly routinely collected surveillance indicators and the comments of the SHA and the local authority's overview and scrutiny committee. PCTs and their partner organisations must demonstrate that they have considered different needs and inequalities in respect of area, socioeconomic group, ethnicity, gender, disability, age, faith and sexual orientation. An inspection visit is made if there is reason for concern about a PCT not meeting the standards. If a PCT fails to satisfy the Healthcare Commission, it must produce an improvement plan and, if performance remains a serious issue, the Department of Health will intervene directly to manage the PCT.

The stronger focus on health inequalities in the planning framework means that PCTs are expected to work jointly with their local authorities, and that this work is reflected in LDPs. PCTs must agree their LDPs with their SHAs, and the plans include information used by the Department of Health to monitor targets. The Spearhead Group of PCTs have three-year trajectories for the trend each is expected to achieve in improving the health of their local populations at substantially faster rates than nationally, closing the gaps with the England average. They must assess progress for the range of issues where action is needed, demonstrate where actions are having the intended effect, and identify measures to tackle issues where progress is not going to plan. Only the Spearhead PCTs are assessed by the Healthcare Commission for their performance in narrowing health inequalities. Non-Spearhead PCTs, which are 80% of all PCTs, are required to reduce health inequalities within their local area by narrowing the gap in all-age all-cause mortality, but this is assessed as part of their LAAs. Both Spearhead and non-Spearhead PCTs should address health inequalities *within* their areas, but this is not performance assessed by the Healthcare Commission because the focus of the Department of Health policy is on narrowing the life expectancy gap between Spearheads and the England average. It is, however, part of what is expected by GO assessments of LSPs receiving NRF and is being incorporated into LAAs and their assessment by GOs in non-Spearhead areas. Closing gaps between neighbourhoods and between groups within the LSP area is expected to be a focus for programmes and performance measures in local NR strategies and LAAs.

The PCT's Director of Public Health (DPH) is responsible for ensuring that services target inequalities. 'Health equity audits' are meant to drive this and are mandatory for all PCTs in England. These are self-assessment and planning tools used to compare service provision with need, and to guide changes in services aimed at making demonstrable impacts on inequalities. One example is a recent health equity audit of CHD by the County Durham and Tees Valley Public Health Network. This compared for each PCT in the region the relative gaps across electoral wards in mortality from CHD with the relative gaps in the elective admission rate for CHD (Low and Low, 2006). In all PCTs, the relative gap in mortality between deprived and affluent wards was greater than the relative gap in admissions, indicating an inequity in provision and a need to achieve a greater rate of access in the deprived wards.

Health equity audits should involve the LSP and can consider wider determinants of health as well as NHS services. However, because of pressure to meet the 2010 health inequalities targets, the focus of these plans is on improving access to, and outcomes from, NHS services. This is where the quickest gains are regarded as achievable, an issue discussed further below. The longer-term perspective on wider determinants of health is not absent, and informs much of *Choosing Health* (DH, 2004a), for which LDPs are key mechanisms for implementation. But the government is looking for tangible progress in narrowing health inequalities that can deliver the measurable and relatively short-term improvements that have been achieved by the performance management of waiting lists.

The role of local authorities and Health Impact Assessment

It is local authorities that have the most potential at a local level to influence the wider determinants of health, and their role in the health inequalities strategy has been strengthened. The performance of local authorities in England and Wales is reviewed by the Audit Commission through an inspection exercise called Comprehensive Performance Assessment (CPA). From 2005/06 CPAs have been extended to include assessing local authorities on their corporate performance in creating healthier communities and tackling health inequalities. Local authorities have to demonstrate how the health of the local population is improving as a result of their activities and what special measures are taken to reach the most vulnerable groups. CPAs will also assess how well the local authority works in partnership with other statutory agencies, in the health field mainly the local NHS but also voluntary agencies and groups representing people who are vulnerable or hard to reach due to literacy, disability or other barriers. Health is one of five shared priority themes that have been agreed nationally between local and central government in England as part of LAAs (more details about these themes can be found at www.idea-knowledge.gov.uk). The Audit Commission and the Healthcare Commission work collaboratively on assessing local performance across local government and the local NHS, with a common focus on the public health standards. This then contributes to the Healthcare Commission's performance assessments and ratings of the local NHS, and the Audit Commission's assessments of local authorities.

Under the 'healthier communities and older people' shared priority theme, local councils are expected to lead in developing effective LSPs and working with partners in the locality to understand and respond to the wider determinants of health locally. They are expected to use audits and performance indicators, involving local people in the process and responding to their priorities. The CPA working group on this theme has identified outcomes and key interventions that can be used as evidence of activity on the ground (see www.communities.gov.uk). These include, for example, improving opportunities for taking exercise and eating healthily, integrating services and improving support for families and older people, meeting the decent homes standard, tackling fuel poverty and improving the take-up of benefits. The inspections look for evidence of achievement and judgements are based on level descriptors. Thus, at level 2 a council will be able to point to improvement in locally agreed short-term indicators for improving health. At level 3 the council is also expected to be able to demonstrate how a longer-term impact on health and life expectancy is being achieved.

In England, LAAs are taking the performance-managed integration of local public services to a new phase. They will be rolled out to all areas from April 2007, and are expected to deliver the objectives of the local Sustainable Community Strategy and the local PSA targets. The 'healthier communities and older people' block is the main focus for health improvement and is expected to link with the PCT's LDP. LAAs should bring health improvement and health inequalities to the forefront of 'community planning'. But as with local PSAs, their strategic focus may seem remote to local residents.

One way to bridge these strategic and neighbourhood levels is through 'neighbourhood management'. This way of working aims to make local services more responsive to local needs at a population scale of around 5,000 to 15,000 residents. In England, the approach has been piloted through a national initiative that started in 2001 and has received a positive evaluation (SQW Ltd, 2006). Estimated to add about £20 per resident annually to local public spending, Neighbourhood Management impacts on the planning and delivery of mainstream public services in a number of ways. One of these is a neighbourhood dimension to performance assessment using service-level agreements (SLAs). These are negotiated agreements between a representative body of local residents and organisations providing local services, with specific outcome targets. Used well, they can join up making service improvements at a neighbourhood level with the contribution of these services to meeting floor targets at the local strategic level. They have been most successful in respect of local policing levels and standards for local environmental services, but have potential to extend into health, especially with the development of health care commissioning by local primary care practices. Indeed, the extent to which neighbourhood SLAs expand will be a test of how far local public bodies are prepared to tie their strategies and budgets into neighbourhood-level agreements.

There is also an issue in an audit culture that is becoming increasingly driven by assessment based on the views of users and the public that the strategic focus will shift downstream to the frontline services that are the main concern of local residents. It is easier to relate to whether a neighbourhood has an easily accessible primary care practice, for example, than to how non-health care services can narrow health inequalities. Both are important but the former is downstream and about treating illness while the latter is upstream and about preventing ill-health.

Health Impact Assessment (HIA) is a method that has been used to evaluate the upstream contribution to health of non-health services and to involve the public in the process (Ardern, 2004). An HIA of Liverpool's housing strategy has demonstrated how the process can also contribute to local policy development (Liverpool City Council et al, 2004). The LSP's Strategic Housing Partnership first commissioned a 'rapid HIA' of the city's Strategic Housing Statement in 2001. This was a scoping exercise, following which a full HIA was commissioned to investigate housing topics that appeared to be most important to the health of the city's residents. A significant risk identified by the HIA was lead in tap water. A subsequent recommendation that removal of lead piping should been incorporated into Liverpool's decent homes target for 2010 was accepted by the City Council's Cabinet. The HIA moved this issue up the agenda for housing improvements, both in the social and private housing sectors. Another significant risk area was construction, for both workers and residents. The HIA identified how demolition work could leave surrounding houses exposed and vulnerable to crime and fly-tipping. Without open communication with residents as part of the redevelopment process, stress and anxiety were likely outcomes (see also Thomas et al's, 2005, study of how residents' stress was significantly raised by housing regeneration in Manchester). Mitigation measures were recommended to ensure site safety and minimise dust and noise.

HIAs should be democratic processes that involve those affected by policies and proposals. In Liverpool, a special effort was made to involve children and young people in areas where a lot of housing clearance was planned. 'Planning for real' and 'priority search' exercises were carried out with primary school children, and street-corner work with teenagers brought them into the process. HIAs can also bring in professionals from outside the health service by assessing how they can be better integrated into a whole system. Liverpool's HIA led to the City Council's environmental health officers widening their role beyond inspecting and enforcing private sector housing standards to providing advice to tenants on safety, other services and benefits. Closer working between environmental health officers, housing professionals and social services was also achieved.

HIAs can be carried out at a range of scales. The Liverpool HIA was fairly large scale and involved a high degree of participation over 18 months. It cost £20,000 plus about a third of the time of three NHS public health professionals during the exercise. As well as assessing health impact, this HIA provided a strategic framework for focusing both funding and effort to tackle upstream causes of health inequality. The approach can also be applied downstream to the health services themselves, with a new hospital the focus of a recent HIA in Liverpool. While just about anything could be assessed, the Liverpool experience is that the biggest contribution of HIA is to policies or programmes that are large scale, of strategic and public concern, commit significant spending, and when the impacts are not known but are likely to be observable and either measurable or have qualitative descriptors (Ardern, 2004).

Local authorities in the UK are now expected to consider across all their services how they can contribute to reducing health inequalities, from planning and transport to housing, trading standards and education. This includes a very wide range of responsibilities: a few examples are creating safe routes for pedestrians and cyclists, enforcing housing and food safety standards, providing play areas and opportunities for physical activity and sport, and working with PCTs and local GPs on exercise referral schemes. Joint projects are becoming more common, such as basing primary care services in a new leisure and sport centre. Local authorities also have the power to undertake scrutiny exercises of health services and health issues in their areas. These exercises typically involve scoping an issue such as fuel poverty or smoking and its impact on health, reviewing the effectiveness of services in tackling the issue, and making recommendations for improvements (see www.cfps.org.uk).

Local authorities have a particularly important role in prevention. Many of the resources of health care systems are used to cope with problems that are preventable. Three types of preventative intervention are relevant: *primary prevention*, whereby action is taken to prevent the onset of a disease or an accident, such as immunisation or promoting exercise to reduce obesity; *secondary prevention*, whereby intervention occurs on the basis of early detection and treatment of the disease or risk factors associated with it, such as screening for cervical cancer or for high blood pressure or cholesterol levels; and *tertiary prevention*, which seeks to minimise the impact of a disease by minimising the disability associated with it through rehabilitation or surgery for example. Local authorities have most potential in primary prevention, but there are advantages in this being delivered within national frameworks that enable both comparison of performance and the exchange of good practice.

An example is the UK government's current road traffic accident target to cut child accidents by 50% by 2010 compared to the average for 1994-98. It is one of three casualty reduction targets set out in the government's road safety strategy, *Tomorrow's Roads: Safer for Everyone* (DETR, 2000). The performance indicator is children under 16 years of age killed or seriously injured in a road accident as a pedestrian, cyclist or car passenger. The main issue is child pedestrian casualties, where the UK's record is poorer than many other European countries. An important approach to planning in relation to a target is to analyse trends and underlying drivers in order to plan interventions that represent a credible means to meet the target. The 2010 child road traffic accident target is expressed as a trajectory of decline from 6,860 children killed or seriously injured in 1994-98 to a target of 3,430 in 2010. Progress towards the target can be monitored by plotting the actual trend against the planned trend up to the most recent time for which data are available. Projecting forward the actual trend enables the extent of any deviation from the planned trend to be determined. This includes looking at the actual annual reduction in a given year compared to the average annual rate of reduction needed to keep on the trajectory, a type of exercise known as 'trajectory planning'.

Analysis of the problem reveals that boys appear to be at almost twice the risk of an accident when walking as girls, and for both sexes the risk of an accident increases with age, so that it is the 8-15 age group that is most at risk (DfT, 2002). Most casualties by far occur on built-up roads and accidents are more likely to take place close to the child's home rather than school. There is also a time dimension: child pedestrian casualties are highest on Fridays and Saturdays and during the summer, when accidents are more likely to occur in the evening. Children in the lowest socioeconomic group are five times more likely to die in a pedestrian road traffic accident than children in the highest group. There is a strong geographical relationship with deprivation, possibly because children from low-income households tend to live in neighbourhoods close to busy roads in areas with few safe play areas. There is also evidence that children from some BME groups may be more at risk than white children living in the same area. Cross-national comparative research points to exposure as the main reason why the UK's child pedestrian fatality rates are higher than those in some other countries. British children spend a similar amount of time walking as their peers in France and the Netherlands, but they make fewer road crossings using designated crossings, spend more time on busy main roads, and are less likely to have an adult with them.

This analysis informs the priorities for action set out as part of the government's road safety strategy in England, Scotland and Wales. Additional funding has been allocated to local authorities for schemes such as 20mph zones and associated traffic calming, safe crossings and child pedestrian training in schools. A research programme continues to investigate areas where understanding is more limited. Most local authorities have local PSAs with the government to improve road safety and demonstrate delivery. Since 2002, the Department for Transport itself has been subject to a PSA to pursue road safety targets and tackle the much higher incidence of serious accidents in deprived areas. The Dealing with Disadvantage initiative aims at integrating road safety measures into local partnership working across transport, education, health and social services users in order to meet the PSA (DfT, 2004). This initiative is also expected to benefit older road users. It has targeted additional funds at 15 local authorities with high rates of deprivation, with the aim of evaluating the approaches taken and developing best practice for other authorities. Government guidance also requires all local authorities to investigate whether they have a road safety problem related to social disadvantage and, if so, to address it and report on progress.

Implementation of the road safety strategy is led by local authorities working with the police, schools and voluntary bodies. Local authorities are required to prepare child road safety audits, which collate and analyse local casualty data, set out a programme to address the issue with local targets, and monitor the results. Demonstration projects to develop good practice have also been promoted. The issue lends itself to HIA as the interactions that lead to accidents are complex and, as discussed in Chapter Two, pedestrian casualties on the roads are emergent outcomes of causal combinations of type of person, type of road and time of day.

Partnerships, whole systems and targets

The child road casualty rate is one of the key performance indicators against which NR areas are monitored, and there has been a gradual closing of the gap between the rate for NR areas and the national average over the past few years. LSPs receiving NRF operate in a performance management regime overseen by their regional GO, but they do not deliver targets directly. They have the important but somewhat difficult task of meeting NR targets through the delivery of their partner organisations, particularly delivering improvements for the most disadvantaged groups and neighbourhoods.

Although there has been a strong tendency for NRF to be used to fund projects that map closely onto disadvantage, the main purpose of NRF is to facilitate a bending of mainstream programmes by experimenting with new ways of delivering services, rather than just adding further, short-term activities. One of the most significant structural changes LSPs can achieve in this respect is the pooling of resources between agencies, either budgets or human or physical resources, to achieve a bigger impact on what needs to be done to meet a common priority or target. The main innovations have been the joint commissioning of care services for both adults and children by local authority social services and PCTs, but there is potential for integration beyond the health and social care dimension.

LSPs receiving allocations from the NRF are required to have a local NR strategy conforming to SMART principles (specific, measurable, achievable, realistic and time-related). Most LSPs incorporate their NR strategy within their Community Strategy. Their annual report on performance to their regional GO is required to review service delivery by assessing progress against national and local targets, self-assessing partnership working and management, and presenting an improvement plan for the next 12 months. As well as establishing accountability for the work of the LSP and its spending of NRF, this process is meant to build capacity among partner agencies, enabling them to better meet their own targets and tackle cross-cutting issues more effectively. In other words, the ambition for LSPs is that the whole is greater than the sum of its parts.

This is difficult to achieve in practice, largely because the separate agencies still have their own priorities and targets to meet, which can divert energy away from partnership working if meeting these imperatives is regarded as most effectively done within the agency's own boundaries. Two approaches, which have a high profile in the NR strategy, offer solutions to this: making intelligent and shared use of data, and targeting. Both approaches have moved centre stage in how LSPs are performance assessed by their regional GOs. The NRF allocations for the period 2006/07 to 2007/08 announced in July 2005 were indicative rather than final, to establish a link between LSP performance and NRF allocations. A key element of the approach is regional GO assessments of LSPs and each floor target area using a 'traffic lights' system. LSPs assessed as amber/red must demonstrate that they have a robust improvement plan and the capacity to deliver it before NRF is released.

The level of detailed analysis involved in meeting these requirements can be illustrated by considering the 2005 *Performance Management Process Report* by the Middlesbrough Partnership (www.middlesbroughpartnership.org.uk). Under a scheme designed to share best practice across local government, Middlesbrough Council was awarded 'Beacon status' by the government in 2002 for its work on NR. The performance report begins by reviewing progress against the three national health floor targets for the NR strategy – female life expectancy, male life expectancy and the conception rate of 15- to 17-year-olds. There was a slight improvement in male life expectancy and teenage conceptions were declining on target. Female life expectancy, however, appeared to have declined between 2001 and

2003. The report comments that this should improve given local survey evidence that lifestyle factors including smoking, diet and exercise were improving (although alcohol consumption was increasing).

Middlesbrough adopted three local health targets as part of its local NR strategy, all concerning lifestyle factors. These are measured using a biennial town-wide survey. Local survey data enable the LSP to analyse variations within the town, and the report focuses on the gap between the neighbourhoods designated as priorities and receiving NRF allocations and the rest of the town (these data were used for the analysis of smoking discussed in Chapter Two). Smoking rates in the NRF areas declined from 43% to 35% between the 2001 and 2003 surveys, closing the gap with the rest of Middlesbrough from 11% to 8% against a 2006 target of 7.6%. Although heavy alcohol consumption increased between the two surveys across the town, the gap declined from 2% to 0.1%, against a target of completely closing the gap by 2006. Only 2003 data are available for physical exercise and this shows regular exercise rates better in NRF areas than in the rest of Middlesbrough, at 33% regularly taking exercise compared to 31% in the rest of the town.

While these data indicate progress in the right direction against incremental targets, they are from samples and the exercise findings are certainly not conclusive about any difference between NRF areas and the rest of the town because of sampling error. The alcohol target is almost met but as a result of consumption apparently increasing faster in the non-NRF areas than the NRF areas. The smoking reduction does appear to represent real progress.

These are all targets that are shared across the Middlesbrough LSP. This sharing of targets across local organisations, which each have a causal contribution to make to an outcome but are only part of a causal combination, defines the 'whole system'. While it is a challenge for LSPs to engage with the degree of complexity this entails, the whole-system approach is influential and one of the best examples is Sure Start. Being a single programme, although a complex intervention, Sure Start benefits from a clarity of purpose and defined responsibilities among partners that are more difficult to achieve in the larger arena of an LSP. The experience of implementation to date, however, has some lessons for the wider NR strategy.

Sure Start is a response to evidence about the importance of early years to a range of outcomes in later life. It targets support at young children and parents. Despite the importance of early years, no one organisation in local or national government had overall responsibility for the under-fives until Sure Start was launched in 1997 to provide integrated services in specific places. It was a whole-system initiative, initially in the most deprived areas, and brought together education, health and social care services at a neighbourhood level, with strong parental and child involvement. The approach is now being mainstreamed for all children and young people as children's trusts in each local authority area. These bring together the local authority, the PCT, voluntary agencies, parents and children, with a strong neighbourhood focus and local delivery in children's centres and extended schools. This broadens out the Sure Start model of integrated local services, outreach, family support and community work with parents.

Children's trusts operate within a single accountability framework despite the different services involved. They are inspected every three years by a JAR that requires education, health, social care and other services to demonstrate outcomes from the work they carry out together for the welfare of children and young people in the local authority area. Targets make outcomes explicit but in doing so can reveal the distance that may exist between policy intent and the realities of local implementation. The national evaluation of Sure Start demonstrates the variability of local conditions and local needs in Sure Start areas, making it very difficult to have a standard national approach to the programme's objectives (Barnes, J. et al, 2005). A study of Sure Start Plus found that some of its objectives and targets are widely regarded as inappropriate and unworkable by local projects (Wiggins et al, 2005). Demands to support pregnant teenagers practically and emotionally left little space to address targets to raise their level of education and improve health-related behaviours such as smoking. Wiggins et al argue that these targets were imposed top-down with no working out of how they would be achieved locally. Better targets would have come from consulting with service providers and users. Some targets also need to be interim measures so that progress can be recognised stage by stage. Attendance at an informal weekly parents group, for example, could be a stage towards re-engaging with formal education.

This illustrates the need to build upwards from the interventions, and their theories of change, to the targets that can be used to monitor progress. Unfortunately this has rarely been done and targets are more often set at a national level and sometimes not even formulated as local targets that have a logical connection with meeting the national target. Different local contexts will mean that the same target reduction is not realistic in every area. Teenage pregnancies are an example: following recognition of this issue as a policy problem with the publication of a Social Exclusion Unit (SEU, 1999) report and comparison with other national trends, reducing teenage pregnancies by 50% by 2010 was introduced as a joint PSA for the Departments of Health and Education and Science, and cascaded down as a 50% reduction target for local government, the local NHS and NRF LSPs. Extra investment was made in the form of a Teenage Pregnancy Local Implementation Grant and the appointment of local teenage pregnancy coordinators, with local monitoring and review conducted by local teenage pregnancy partnership boards accountable to regional teenage pregnancy coordinators and assessment panels, and overall progress monitored by a National Independent Advisory Group.

Figure 6.1 shows that there has been a small downward trend in teenage conception rates in recent years in both NRF and non-NRF areas in England. However, if we contrast two NRF LSPs in one region of England, the North West, the trajectories are very different. Blackpool has seen an already high rate of teenage conceptions rise even further, while Pendle has seen a much faster fall than nationally, taking it well below the NRF average. The teenage pregnancy strategy appears to be succeeding well in Pendle but failing in Blackpool. As discussed in the concluding chapter, an advantage of performance assessment data is the ability to make these comparisons and then dig deeper into the reasons for observed differences. But this means that the targets are likely to need revision as the effects of local context become apparent. The reasons for differences in outcomes will include differences in what programmes are being delivered, differences in how programmes are being delivered, and differences in context. Chapter Five discussed how QCA can be used to explore these factors and identified some contextual factors that appear to be important in affecting teenage conception rates. Targets should therefore reflect these local contextual conditions. This thinking has influenced target setting in some fields, notably school inspections. From September 2005, inspections of schools in England place a strong emphasis on a contextualised measure of student progress that takes into account the impact on students' attainment of factors such as deprivation, ethnicity and mobility as well as prior attainment (see www.ofsted.gov.uk). A lot more work of this kind needs to be undertaken to inform setting targets for NR, and comparing progress in a way that has a realistic connection with the performance that can be expected in a given local context, including health targets.

Figure 6.1: Trends in teenage conception rate

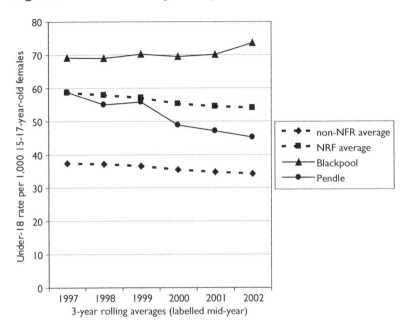

Although much more needs to be done to improve health inequality targeting at a local level, there is no doubt that by bringing health inequalities within the ambit of audit culture changes in priorities and strategies are being engendered. Improving public health and narrowing health inequalities are now recognised as crucial to the effectiveness of the NHS system and managing demands on it from preventable causes of ill-health. This is emphasised in *Choosing Health* (DH, 2004a) and its delivery plan (DH, 2005d), and through the new public health standards that will be used by the Healthcare Commission to review annually the local performance of the NHS in England (Healthcare Commission, 2005b). These standards require health care organisations to work with local authorities, LSPs and other organisations to improve health and narrow health inequalities. Emphasis is placed on running disease prevention and health promotion programmes for nutrition and exercise, smoking, alcohol and substance misuse, and sexually transmitted diseases. Primary care is also being focused more strongly on preventative advice, screening, proactive case finding and early treatment. An important vehicle for this is the Quality and Outcomes Framework (QOF) introduced in 2004 as part of a new NHS contract with GPs across the UK. This rewards GPs financially for achieving clinical and management targets and better services for patients as measured by an array of quality indicators that trigger additional payments.

These are important developments because performance assessment counts in public services: organisational, professional and political reputations, senior jobs and careers, and budgets depend on the outcomes, certainly in the English system. It is an ambitious agenda, with uncertainties, complexities and defects. The QOF, for example, has been criticised for failing to incentivise the right outcomes, especially health gains, and absorbing funds that could be spent on lower-cost and more beneficial preventative measures (Fleetcroft and Cookson, 2006). The expectation that local authorities are community leaders and will take forward the health inequalities agenda through the LSP appears to conflict with the NHS developmental standard that PCTs take the lead role in tackling health inequalities locally. And despite efforts to coordinate NHS and local government inspections, these are still two separate regimes, with the performance management of LSPs adding a third. There are also different approaches to these issues in England, Wales and Scotland, although there is a common emphasis on partnership working, especially between the NHS and local government. In England, there is a stronger performance management approach, extending beyond the NHS to link with the inspection regime for local government, so that there is shared accountability at chief executive levels for making progress with health improvement and inequality targets. The NHS has the lead role, but is expected to work in partnership with local government and community and voluntary organisations to achieve its targets at local level.

For each national health target, the LDP of each PCT is monitored by its SHA along certain 'lines', with criteria specified for signing off the LDP according to performance against these monitoring lines. Each target is linked to commitments made in *Choosing Health* (DH, 2004a) and guidance has been issued by the Department of Health to PCTs about the key interventions and best practice regarded as necessary to meet the target. Table 6.2 illustrates this process for tackling obesity.

What is soon clear from Table 6.2, however, is that, although the PCT is accountable for progress with the obesity target, most of the key interventions require action outside the sphere of the NHS in schools, workplaces and the community. Upstream interventions, though, need to reach large numbers of people to achieve health gains: a reduction of 15,000 people with obesity-related CHD would require reducing the number of people who are obese by one million, clearly

Table 6.2: Planning to tackle obesity

Priority	Tackling obesity
National target	Halt the year-on-year rise in obesity among children by 2010 in the context of a broader strategy to tackle obesity in the population as a whole.
LDP monitoring lines	Childhood obesity. Obesity status among the GP registered population aged 15-75.
Criteria for LDP sign-off	An increase in the number of children and adults with their weight recorded (body mass index). Plans aimed at halting the rise in childhood obesity by 2010. A decrease over time in GP patients with a BMI of 30 or greater. An integrated approach to a broad obesity strategy.
Relevant *Choosing Health* commitments	Development of a comprehensive care pathway for treating obesity. Free school fruit for 4- to 6-year-olds. All schools to have active travel plans by 2010. Health professionals encouraged to use pedometers in clinical practice.
Big wins: key interventions and best practice	Schools: school nurses identifying and helping children at risk. Improved school meals and free fruit. Promoting school sport. Children's travel: action to promote cycling and walking to school. Early years interventions: promoting breastfeeding; promoting healthy lifestyles through Sure Start. Obesity care pathway and support services. Physical activity: promoting physical activity at work, through sport and transport. Diet: more community initiatives to promote fruit and vegetable consumption, targeting disadvantaged areas. Parks and public spaces: promoting greater use for physical activity.

Source: adapted from Neighbourhood Renewal Unit (2005b)

an important target but large in comparison to the downstream gains (NAO, 2001). Because obesity is very difficult to treat clinically the best strategy is increasing physical activity and changing diet. But this is less true of the 2010 targets for heart disease, stroke and cancer, where the emphasis is on treatment and screening, given the potential of medical interventions to achieve reductions in mortality among the large numbers of people already with a disease or at high risk. The health inequality aspect of this medical focus is that of recognising and acting on the higher than average likelihood that people from 'routine and manual' occupational backgrounds will delay consulting their GP, and the lower likelihood of being promptly referred for diagnosis, given treatment or attending screening. Thus, despite the importance of wider determinants of health outside the sphere of the NHS, 'The work of the NHS is absolutely crucial to addressing health inequalities and, like many other services, if it does not pro-actively deliver prevention and health services in ways which will narrow inequalities the default position is that it will probably widen them' (DH, 2005c, p 1). Hence the emphasis on extending the target-setting and performance management approach that has characterised tackling waiting lists for treatment to the more complex 'wicked issue' of health inequalities.

Within the NHS, most progress is regarded as possible through secondary prevention. This is reflected, for example, in the significant upward trend in levels of treated and controlled high blood pressure cases in the population (NHS Health and Social Care Information Centre, 2005). Although McKeown (1979) argued that health care services contributed very little to the major declines in mortality that occurred in developed countries from the mid-19th to mid-20th centuries, effective and timely health care has an important role to play in preventing deaths from the chronic diseases. These have increased in prevalence considerably since the 1960s when McKeown was writing. This has focused attention on avoidable mortality that is amenable to health care, and a great deal of progress was made during the 1980s with improved health care interventions, contributing to rising life expectancy across the countries of the European Union. The main impact was from declining infant mortality but in some countries, including the UK, reductions in deaths among middle-aged people contributed at least as much to this rising life expectancy (Nolte and McKee, 2004). Progress faltered during the 1990s, however, especially in northern Europe where there was by this time less scope for improving infant mortality compared to the higher starting point of countries such as Greece and Portugal.

These health care improvements include new drugs and technologies as well as the better organisation of services, such as multidisciplinary stroke units and integrated screening programmes. In the US, 72% of the decline in deaths from ischaemic heart disease during the 1980s is estimated as due to secondary prevention, compared to a quarter estimated as attributable to primary prevention, pointing to a key role for medical care (Nolte and McKee, 2004). However, Unal et al (2005) contradict this US evidence with models using data from England and Wales. Mortality from CHD fell by 54% between 1981 and 2000 and they estimate that approximately half of this large fall was due to primary prevention, which they defined as reductions in the three major risk factors for CHD in people without recognised disease – smoking, cholesterol and blood pressure. This is a fourfold larger reduction in deaths than those they estimate as attributable to secondary prevention. The difference with the US may reflect different definitions of primary and secondary prevention, but the UK evidence points to the need to prioritise population-wide tobacco control and healthier diets, and not to overplay the contribution of secondary prevention. Lung cancer presents an even stronger case for primary prevention – particularly cutting smoking prevalence – because treatment is often not successful once the disease starts.

The effectiveness of primary prevention chimes with evidence that geographical differences in the quality or quantity of health care in developed countries appear to make little difference to mortality rates for diseases amenable to medical treatment (Mackenbach and Bakker, 2002). These rates vary significantly between places, although this is largely explained by associations with ethnicity and social class. The apparent lack of a relationship between health care provision and amenable mortality, but a strong relationship with social class and ethnicity, may be due to the direct effects of living and working conditions on risk or to differences in the utilisation of care and the quality of care received. Nolte and McKee (2004) argue that, with gains in life expectancy from rising living standards becoming harder to achieve because such a large proportion of the population enjoy generally healthy living conditions, health care services have an important role to play in achieving further gains in life expectancy. This is not the same thing, however, as reducing health inequality. Adverse material conditions in the home, neighbourhood or workplace, and low income, remain problems for significant minorities of people in countries like the UK and the US. This is not to deny that health care is an important part of the picture and has a key role in reducing health inequality, but preventive programmes beyond health care remain particularly important.

Health inequality strategy as a direction of travel

It might be thought to undermine the rationale for this book to consider the *lack* of progress to date with closing the health divide in the UK, given my general support for the strategies that are in place. But just as there is more that can be done to improve these strategies, and particularly their engagement with key drivers of change, there is also a need to allow time for the tide to turn. These are strategies that need long-term commitment. For as long as the UK has governments in power that regard health inequalities as an important issue, the health inequality strategies now look established for the long term. There is currently a lot of focus on the 2010 targets but these are milestones and not end-points.

The NR strategy is less certain. The current phase of funding ends in 2008 and the strategy, along with health and other public spending generally, will have to establish its claim to a much more slowly expanding public expenditure cake. The NR strategy was established as a short-life initiative because its aim is to mainstream service improvements and new ways of working. There is not the evidence yet, however, that the foot can be taken off the accelerator. The UK's deprived neighbourhoods still need major national programmes focused on closing the gap with the rest of the country.

The latest data for both life expectancy and infant mortality show a continuing trend of widening inequality (DH, 2005a). Between 1997–99 and 2001–03, the gap in life expectancy between the fifth of local authorities with the lowest life expectancy and England as a whole increased by 2% for males and 5% for females. In 2001–03, the infant mortality rate among 'routine and manual' occupational groups was 19% higher than for the total population, compared to 13% in 1997–99 (despite, like life expectancy, an overall improvement). On the plus side, a range of other indicators suggests that it is reasonable to expect these gaps to begin closing if current programmes are sustained. In particular, progress with reducing deaths from heart disease has been good, including in disadvantaged areas, although with the recent improvements attributed not to the reduction of the underlying causes of circulatory diseases but to increased prescribing of statins and better stroke treatment. There is also evidence of some improvement with cancers. In the longer term, the substantial improvements that are occurring in housing, in reducing fuel poverty and in young people's educational achievement should feed through into future health improvements. Other indicators have not so far improved, although they are all targeted by government programmes. These include fruit and vegetable consumption, physical exercise and homelessness. The availability of GPs is also a concern. The number of GPs has increased since 2002, including in deprived areas, but by 2004 around half of PCTs in the fifth most deprived areas of England were more than 10% below the national average level of GP provision, compared to only a third in 2002.

Neighbourhoods have attracted attention both for the assessment of health status and for action and monitoring to improve health status. Geographical variation in health outcomes is the main reason for this policy focus. Figures 6.2 and 6.3 show the variation in life expectancy at birth for men and women at the scale of district council areas in England, using data from the Office for National Statistics. This is graphed against a measure of multiple deprivation, the IMD average score for 2004. The graphs show a strong negative relationship between life expectancy and deprivation. Two points are noteworthy. Firstly, although England has health inequality targets that are about reducing the gap between the worst 20% of areas and the national average, this average summarises a range of values rather than being in any way typical. The targeted 20% are at the bottom of a gradient. Secondly, the bottom 20% of areas by deprivation includes about half of all people on low incomes, but this total is falling (Palmer et al, 2005). Although health inequalities are showing little improvement so far, they are affecting less people 'at the bottom'. In 2003/04 there were 12 million people in Britain – about one in five – living on incomes below the relative poverty line of 60% or less of the national median household income. This is nearly two million less than in the early 1990s (Palmer et al, 2005). It is important not to exaggerate this point as the level of relative poverty is still nearly twice what it was in the late 1970s. Falling unemployment has contributed to the recent decline but there has been a rise in the number of 'working poor' and the UK stands out by European standards regarding the proportion of children living in workless households.

Just as targeting areas will not do on its own to tackle deprivation, targeting deprivation will not reach all areas or people where ill-health is a problem. The relationships between deprivation and life expectancy in Figures 6.2 and 6.3 are strong but there is quite a lot of 'unexplained' variation, with a range in life expectancies for similar IMD values. This is even more the case at a smaller geographical scale. Figures 6.4 and 6.5 show for males and females respectively the relationships between life expectancy and deprivation at ward level in Hounslow, North London. The data are from the London Health Observatory (http://www.lho.org.uk). The graphs include the 95% confidence intervals to illustrate how at this scale there is a substantial margin of

Figure 6.2: Male life expectancy by deprivation, English local authorities

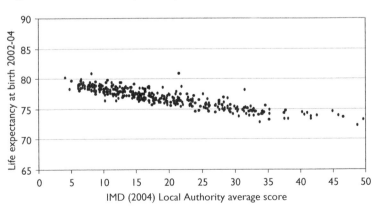

Figure 6.3: Female life expectancy by deprivation, English local authorities

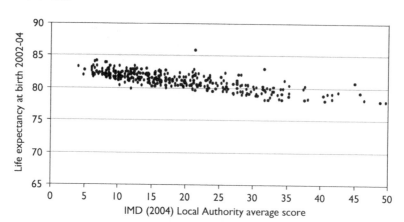

error involved in estimating life expectancy. For males, there are five wards with relatively low deprivation and high life expectancies, but for the other wards the pattern is not very clear. For females, there is no apparent relationship between deprivation and life expectancy. If wards are used as a basis for targeting health interventions, there are four or five wards that could be candidates for these measures, but they are not the most deprived. Analysis at a smaller scale of Super Output Areas might reveal a stronger relationship with deprivation, but the confidence intervals then become even wider. Alternatively, there could be a combination of neighbourhood compositional and contextual factors behind these uneven geographies of life expectancy in Hounslow.

Although the geography of deprivation is very much part of the larger picture, at the local level more is going on that needs to be

Figure 6.4: Male life expectancy by deprivation, Hounslow wards

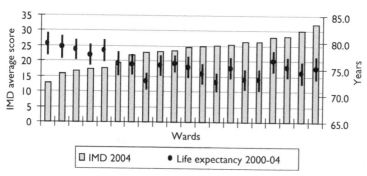

Figure 6.5: Female life expectancy by deprivation, Hounslow wards

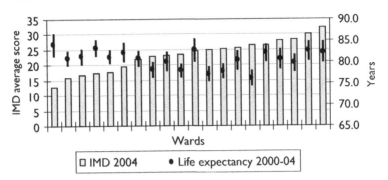

taken into account. This was the main message of Chapter Four in looking at neighbourhood attributes and their causal combinations. Chapter Five and this chapter have extended this to considering the performance of local services and of whole areas. The Spearhead areas, for example, vary significantly in the progress that is being made with contributing to the national life expectancy targets. A recent review by the Prime Minister's Delivery Unit concluded that this reflects differences in the strength of local leadership and focus on the targets, as well as the importance of secondary prevention among people in their fifties and sixties (NRU briefing, January 2006). The review is likely to see all Spearheads given targets recast as models of the progress they can be expected to achieve, based on evidence of the impact of interventions such as statins prescribing and smoking cessation services on the local pattern of premature mortality.

Figures 6.6 and 6.7 show the extent of progress with closing gaps for three of the health floor targets across the 21 LSPs in North West England that receive NRF. Hyndburn has seen a narrowing of the gap in premature mortality from circulatory diseases by 30 deaths as measured by the standardised mortality rate. Burnley, on the other hand, has seen this gap widen by 16 deaths. There are two points in particular to note from these graphs: the variable 'performance' of areas, which appears to show no relationship to differences between them in deprivation, and the differences by floor targets – some LSP areas are doing well for one target but not for the other. There is potential for these areas to learn from each other, especially to explore whether there are particular interventions, or combinations of interventions, that are associated with those LSPs where inequalities are narrowing.

Figure 6.6: Relative change in circulatory diseases mortality at ages under 75, 1999-2003, North West LSPs

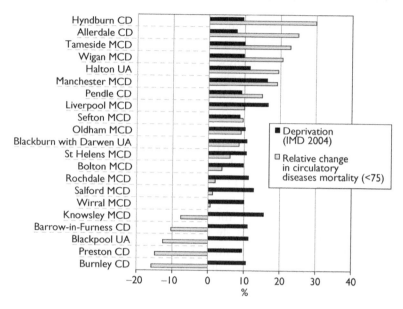

Figure 6.7: Relative change in cancers mortality at ages under 75, 1999-2003, North West LSPs

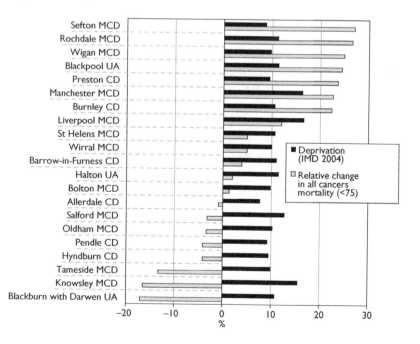

Health inequalities and the performance management culture

All the main agencies providing services to neighbourhoods have a variety of targets which they are expected to meet to justify their public funding. For a PCT these targets currently include reducing deaths from cancer and heart disease, and inequalities in these death rates; better management of blood pressure and cholesterol by GPs; improving cancer treatment; reducing adult smoking prevalence and smoking during pregnancy; increasing breastfeeding; tackling childhood obesity; reducing teenage pregnancies and improving access to sexual health services; and improving mental health, including reducing suicide rates. Each PCT's LDP sets out how it expects to meet these nationally set targets and priorities as well as locally agreed objectives. PCTs know where they need to get to and when, and they must report on progress regularly. Priorities are improving treatment, especially early diagnosis and quicker treatment following diagnosis, and tackling risk factors, especially obesity (including poor diet and physical inactivity) and smoking, which are common risk factors for both of the major causes of death in the UK – cancers and circulatory diseases. PCTs are expected to provide leadership together with the local authority and across a range of other organisations to drive concerted action on health inequalities, both through their LDPs and beyond NHS services to the health impact of local government and other services.

A key consideration is to ensure that health improvement programmes do not increase gaps in health inequalities by having a greater impact on the health of better-off people, who not only face lower risks of becoming ill than poorer people but are also often more likely to be diagnosed early and survive following diagnosis. Cancer screening programmes, for example, need to compensate for social and individual differences in accessing them with both 'outreach' and 'inreach' measures (Chiu, 2003).

A distinctive feature of recent developments in English policy to tackle health inequalities is performance management to provide transparent data on progress and hold national and local bodies to account. England, Scotland and Wales have different 'audit cultures' in this respect, and have also taken different paths in responding to health inequalities since devolution in 1998. Greer (2006) argues that this reflects the different policy communities of these countries, although there is some evidence now of convergence, especially as Scotland and Wales identify a need for local comparative data that was neglected earlier due to political opposition to performance league tables (Audit Scotland, 2005; Scottish Executive, 2005; Welsh Assembly Government, 2005; Audit General for Wales, 2006). Performance management based on comparison has been credited with reducing waiting times for treatment in England, and the Healthcare Commission has recently argued that targets have driven up standards in many treatment and preventative services that are not apparent for services without targets (Healthcare Commission, 2005a).

It is not clear that a similar approach of setting targets and publishing outcomes at the level of individual organisations will have the same effect on tackling an issue as complex and cross-cutting as health inequalities. It certainly exacerbates the issue of establishing a causal chain from interventions to outcomes. The English reforms of public services inspection embrace narrowing health inequalities so that this is 'seen to matter' in a system of rewards and sanctions, a change that is occurring within the wider framework of joining up inspections of public bodies, establishing an outcomes focus and reducing their administrative burden (DH, 2004b; Healthcare Commission et al, 2004; Bundred, 2005). While both Scotland and Wales use data about health inequalities to assess local performance, the inspection regimes are lighter and currently lack the cross-cutting elements of the English system, despite the strong emphasis in both countries on partnership working. Recently, the government-commissioned Lyons Inquiry has argued that the number of centrally imposed and inspected targets in England is excessive and that they need to be reduced and better focused (Lyons, 2006). Lyons argues that this is needed to create more space for local participation, responsiveness and innovation, and that local variation in some services should be less constrained by central targets.

Performance assessment would seem to be an enduring feature of the new regulatory state but is undergoing reform to steer more and row less (Hood, 2002). In England, new vehicles are being put in place that focus on outcomes but also engage with the cross-cutting character of wicked issues. For health inequalities these include LSPs, PSA targets, shared priorities, LAAs and JARs. Failure to make progress with shared health inequality priorities will threaten a poorer assessment for both a local authority and a local PCT because both agencies will be expected to share and deliver on this outcome.

These changes in England are taking place within a national audit regime based on top-down performance measurement with strong managerial incentives, and both SHAs and GOs are likely to continue to exercise considerable power over how localities move forward with the agenda. This is potentially in conflict with the learning rather than regulatory culture needed to tackle wicked issues: it may work with waiting times but health inequalities present a different challenge. There remain risks that more politically sensitive targets such as waiting lists will take priority and that local authorities will not fully engage given the many other pressures on them to meet performance targets. There are still problems with attempting to assess outcomes over time periods that are too short and to evaluate the effectiveness of interventions when these may be different, or differently implemented, across diverse local contexts. A further risk is that encountered by the HAZs: shifts in government priorities centrally forcing changes locally so that there is no sustained focus on issues (Barnes et al, 2003).

There is a danger of this occurring as the 2010 life expectancy targets approach. This is leading PCTs to turn their attention to interventions for those who already have, or are at high risk of having, one of the major killer diseases. The focus is on clinical services and treatments, especially for circulatory diseases and cancers. It is also on the over-50s, where deaths contribute three quarters of the gap in life expectancy between the most deprived areas and the national average. Within this timeframe, effective strategies are likely to be interventions such as treatment with statins, anti-obesity drugs and anti-hypertensives. The importance of these downstream measures should not be underestimated if they result in significant reconfigurations of local services and spending. Sheffield, for example, has achieved a faster decline in heart disease in its most deprived areas than across the city as a whole by improving how well secondary prevention is targeted on social and ethnic inequalities (DH, 2005c). But they may detract from other strategies and public policy interventions focusing on primary prevention and its longer timescale upstream.

It is upstream that the causes of wicked problems lie but their complexity intensifies what can be described as the 'black box' problem: the relationship between an action and an outcome is problematic due to problems of interdependencies and causal attribution (University of Birmingham, 1999; Kavanagh and Richards, 2001; Hudson and Henwood, 2002). A command-and-control approach to performance managing such issues is unlikely to relate well to their nature as 'a constellation of linked problems embedded in the fabric of the communities in which they occur', and stakeholders grappling with wicked issues often bring to them different interpretations, values and goals (Kreuter et al, 2004, p 441). Even when particular interventions are known to have an effect likely to narrow health inequalities, there can be disagreement and uncertainty about the merits of alternative options. For example, a PCT will be tempted to maximise funding for the secondary prevention measures discussed above, but could instead share funding with a local authority to fund benefit take-up campaigns or help with finding and sustaining employment. Assessing these options is very difficult because the relationship between what partner agencies in a locality do and whether the gap in life expectancy or teenage pregnancies narrows is unlikely to be straightforward. It is not a mechanical or linear relationship but one of complexity and asymmetry. This complexity arises from the emergent outcomes of interaction, and these are contingent, contextual and difficult to predict in detail (such as doing A will achieve B).

Evidence from the Best Value regime in local government suggests that the principle of learning and improvement was often lost because of a preoccupation with meeting individual service targets (Rashman and Radnor, 2005). Performance assessment is ideally part of an explicit learning framework for a complex adaptive system, whether a local authority, PCT or LSP. Plsek and Greenhalgh (2001, p 625) define a complex adaptive system as 'a collection of individual agents with freedom to act in ways that are not always totally predictable, and whose actions are interconnected so that one agent's actions changes the context for other agents'. This behaviour gives rise to important features of such systems: context dependency, feedback loops, emergent non-linear change, and unintended consequences (Chapman, 2004). An example is smoking cessation. A mechanistic approach to missing a smoking cessation target would be for the PCT to increase funding for cessation services. This reflects a linear model of change: more spending on these services produces a decline in smokers. However, there is now considerable evidence that the contexts in which smoking rates are highest are where people are coping with worklessness, very low incomes or poor neighbourhood liveability such as dereliction or crime (see Chapter Two). Higher spending on cessation services may have the unintended consequence of widening the gap in smoking rates between people living with these conditions and others who are more motivated to respond to health promotion messages. A more successful strategy may be to focus the resources of both the PCT and local authority on reducing levels of worklessness and crime in the most deprived areas, creating the conditions in which people consider it worth investing in their future health by giving up smoking.

Plsek (2001) and Chapman (2004) propose a number of principles that can inform this kind of adaptive systems thinking and which can be summarised as follows:

- learning 'what works' from local innovation and experimentation;
- sharing information and making connections between people;
- creating simple rules for innovation and development that move the system in the right direction, for example avoid actions likely to widen inequalities, even if these are likely to improve health for some;
- evaluating overall system performance with stakeholders as co-evaluators.

Conclusion: the neighbourhood setting and health

The neighbourhood offers a 'midstream' level of intervention for this complex systems approach. It is where experimentation can take place and connections can be made. It is also increasingly seen as a meaningful level of organisation for community and political participation (Mulgan and Bury, 2006). Neighbourhoods can be a setting for targeting case-finding and early treatment, with their focus on the individual, but they are also systems that influence the health-related behaviours of their residents as a group. Physical activity is an important example, particularly the potential of more walkable neighbourhoods to encourage the large group of sedentary people in societies such as the UK to take at least occasional exercise.

In England, 60% of men and 70% of women are not active at the level recommended for health benefits (NRU, 2005b). Interventions such as primary care exercise referral schemes and more time for school sport are important, but the underlying problem is one of 'obesogenic environments' (Health Committee, 2004). Neighbourhoods can be obesogenic if they do not encourage walking on a daily basis, with public transport, shops, health centres and schools within reach by safe and attractive walking routes. Some studies have explored what attributes of a neighbourhood encourage walking, identifying factors such as nearby, large and attractive parks with facilities that encourage active use by multiple users, local shops, removal of traffic, and places to sit (Foster et al, 2004; Pasaogullari and Doratli, 2004; Giles-Corti et al, 2005; Naderi and Raman, 2005).

The existence of local amenities and services is not enough to promote walking if environmental factors discourage it (Giles-Corti and Donovan, 2002). Evidence from a number of international studies points to attributes such as greenery and low levels of litter and graffiti as important in promoting outdoor physical activity (Ellaway et al, 2005). Safety is particularly significant. Shenassa et al (2006) found that a neighbourhood perceived as safe raised the odds of occasional exercise among women by 22%, and of frequent exercise by 40%. Among men the odds of occasional exercise were raised by 39%, although with no effect on frequent exercise. Perception of safety was significantly influenced by the amount of litter and graffiti, and was worse in areas of panel-block housing or multi-family dwellings compared to single-family detached housing. In another study Alexander et al (2005) found that levels of moderate to vigorous physical activity *throughout the day* were substantially higher among adolescents who walked to school. Chapter Three discussed the evidence that walking may slow the progression of dementia. Finally, concerns about neighbourhood safety do not just discourage outdoor physical activity. They may affect utilisation of local services, including health care, an effect that Whitley and Prince (2005) found was most marked among low-income mothers in their North London study.

While these types of study of statistical associations point to the importance of walkable neighbourhoods for health, evaluations of interventions are less common, and economic evaluations are even rarer. Cost–benefit analyses such as that of Sælensminde (2004), which demonstrates the appreciable health cost savings arising from walking and cycle track networks in Norway, are important in securing political commitment.

Evidence, however, can conflict with political or public opinion, and question initiatives in vogue with professionals. 'Food deserts' are an example. These are low-income neighbourhoods where residents have poor access to reasonably priced fruit and vegetables. Many local NR strategies have programmes aimed at this issue. Yet the evidence for the existence of food deserts is mixed. Just improving the provision of fruit and vegetables, even at affordable prices, is complicated by factors such as motivation, family responsibilities and smoking that intervene between the cost and actual consumption of healthy food and a healthy diet (Cummins and Macintyre, 2002; Whelan et al, 2002). Various interventions have sought to improve access to healthy food, from attracting supermarkets to regenerated areas and promoting food co-ops and allotments, to linking kitchen replacements in housing improvement programmes with one-to-one consultation and awareness-raising events to promote healthy cooking (Freeman, 2004). Very few evaluations have been published; one 'before and after' study found that a new superstore located in an area of high deprivation was associated with a 'modest impact' on diet (Wrigely et al, 2003).

Public health evidence still has many gaps and is often not conclusive. One of the reasons for this is the contingency introduced by local context, and part of this context is the 'voice' of local residents and their priorities and preferences. Central targets are needed to compare progress and pose questions about relative performances, but local autonomy and innovation may get crowded out by local managers focusing exclusively on them. Space for local autonomy is needed because experimentation and learning are necessary in every local context given that there are rarely standard models than can credibly link programmes on the ground with meeting targets, whether locally or centrally defined. Local public opinion may also be at odds with strategies that are strongly evidence-based, such as redeploying funds from health care to primary prevention, or with the very principle of narrowing health inequalities rather than improving average health. As the climate shifts to reducing targets further and giving residents and users greater voice, the case for engaging publics with the bigger picture of health inequality and the use, testing and creation of evidence becomes more important. Otherwise, the agenda of reducing inequality represented by the NR and health inequality targets in England could be eclipsed by the agendas of localism and choice in public services. These are not agendas that are necessarily in conflict but they do need strategies that align them, connecting the local and the global. The concluding chapter turns to this issue.

SEVEN

Conclusion: neighbourhoods in the wider picture

Layard (2005), in what I believe is an important book, maps out the 'new science' of happiness, a state associated with, but not the same as, good health. Ultimately, policies for neighbourhoods should be aiming at happy neighbourhoods as well as healthy ones. Step outside the front door and there are things to be happy about rather than things that are troubling or stressful. These may be a job to go to; a place for children to play and teenagers to hang out; neighbours that we trust and spend some time with; contact with nature and trees; an environment that is looked after, reflects well on us and is free from hazards; shops and services that are reachable; participation in decisions that affect us and our neighbourhood; and, above all, a place that we want to be. This does not mean that the neighbourhood necessarily makes a great difference for many of us, but that the more it constrains, stresses or disables us the more likely it is that our health will be damaged. Neighbourhoods, therefore, are a legitimate object of policy. They are systems that among their many inputs may sometimes need policy interventions.

Amin (2002) suggests that we think of places as nodes in networks of relationships that situate practices in space. I have gone further than this to argue that residential places are systems. Amin argues that practices may or may not reinforce local connections so that the place itself has agency. He plays down any idea that places have a special agency in themselves. As nodes of situated practices they are less obviously agents than firms, governments, social movements or other types of organisation. Practices in a place will often have much more significant relationships with networks beyond that place than with the place itself, so 'places are more than what they contain, and what happens in them is more than the sum of localised practices and powers, and actions at other 'spatial scales'' (Amin, 2002, p 395). However, Amin does not deny the significance of proximity and particularity in space, both because levels of government are organised territorially, and because these characteristics engender political and social movements and local action of various kinds. But he reminds us that this action, although situated locally, engages with relational networks beyond any single place.

A frequent criticism of ABIs in social policy has been that they ignore the wider networks of economic and political power that make the real difference to people's lives. Even the argument that the local area is a meaningful level at which to engage people in action to improve health falls foul of Amin's point that people everywhere are engaged in many networks that affect their lives, so why focus on often quite weak and transient local networks? This is the old argument in another guise about territorial communities and non-territorial communities, or communities of interest. The former is still widely used in social policy as an intervention framework. One of the four priorities of the Department of Health's *Tackling Health Inequalities: A Programme for Action* is 'engaging communities and individuals to ensure relevance, responsiveness and sustainability ... strengthening capacity to tackle local problems and pools of deprivation' (DH, 2003, pp 4, 10). Thus the plan calls for 'improved access to public services in disadvantaged communities' (p 4) and 'local solutions for local health inequality problems given that local planners, frontline staff and communities know best what their problems are' (p 5). It recognises other networks, such as national programmes, ethnic communities and 'vulnerable' communities, and does not use the term 'community' in an exclusively spatial way, but endorses the NR strategy with its strong focus on 'deprived neighbourhoods'.

Neighbourhoods do evolve within the overall order and structure of urban society. They are real spaces that change and adapt, and can stand in marked contrast to the abstract 'space' of official and bureaucratic decision making, such as when local residents come into conflict with plans to redevelop their neighbourhood (Blackman, 1991; Taylor, 1999). Neighbourhoods derive their social significance from their proximate status, centred on the home and the most emotional site of lived experience for many people, compared with the remoteness of other systems of governance, production or consumption. Their apparently declining significance in a world of increased mobility, delocalised economic systems and multiple communities of identity and interest is not because they have disappeared. It is because growing complexity means that there are far more spaces in people's lives that form part of their experiences and material existence including, of course, telemediated spaces and cyberspaces.

In *Urban Policy in Practice* I defined 'communities' as 'local populations identifiable from their wider society by a more intense sharing of concerns or by increased levels of interaction' (Blackman, 1995, p 143).

In this book I have taken this further in proposing that these dimensions of geography, identity and behaviour come together not just as nodes in relational networks but as open dynamic systems with emergent properties. They have some organisational coherence as a result of processes of self-organisation, interaction and feedback. Neighbourhoods are open systems because they are bounded environments that create a setting or context for self-organising action that is interactively connected across the neighbourhood boundary with other systems. These boundaries are often fuzzy, fluid and even socially constructed. Yet even as social constructions their effects can be real enough. For most people, asking them whether they live in a good or bad neighbourhood *means* something.

Disadvantaged neighbourhoods are not necessarily 'bad' neighbourhoods. However, poor liveability, problems with antisocial behaviour and poor local services are too often part of the picture in the most deprived areas. The NR strategy includes a commitment to improve public services, and community involvement is seen as a key element. This requires more than sharing information and consultation; community involvement in deprived areas calls for intensive and deliberate engagement with people whose awareness of services may be low and access poor. It is a means of service providers gaining better local knowledge of needs, raising awareness of existing services, and improving services so that they are not just better funded but also more personal and offer choice. This demands a different way of working, and is likely to lead to a need for change in how services are designed and delivered. Therefore, a planning and budgetary commitment to localising decision making so that innovation and flexibility are possible is an important precondition for community involvement that makes a difference. This engagement need not stop at the neighbourhood scale. Indeed, if neighbourhood governance is about enlivening democracy then neighbourhoods should be a platform for engagement with societies and the social patterns and inequalities that influence and sometimes end lives.

Neighbourhoods of engagement

The neighbourhood is where 'things go on' around the home. This is why definitions of 'liveability' tend to relate to what can be seen or heard within comfortable walking distance of the home: the walkable sphere of experience. This is also a shared experience; the neighbourhood is the shared space beyond the front door before somewhere else is reached, and this can give rise to both conflict and collective action. This shared experience extends to a 'joined-up' character to the neighbourhood, and when public services do not join up at neighbourhood level this is regarded as a delivery failure.

Getting this right, therefore, means 'engaging communities' so that what is done is sustainable and co-produced by services and residents. Sustainability will also increasing extend to ecological considerations and to the eco-neighbourhood as a place where power is generated from renewable micro-generation, recycling and local production occurs, and priority is given to jobs and services within reach of walking, cycling or public transport (Rudlin and Falk, 1999). Community development may be needed to build the partnerships to make things happen. This often starts with extra funding for community workers to initiate organised activity, building on any existing organisation, or by seconding professional workers to community development roles, such as health visitors released from individual case work to spend time developing contacts with residents and building up community activities. In Hastings, for example, the Greater Hollington Neighbourhood Management Pathfinder, one of an early wave of Neighbourhood Management initiatives, has included relocating a team of health visitors to an office in one of the area's high-rise blocks of flats, together with a health community development worker (Healthier Neighbourhoods Action Team, 2005). A range of interventions has focused on raising awareness about health, school breakfast clubs, a healthy eating café, a supermarket stroke awareness campaign, after-school and holiday physical activities for children and young people, health walks, and assessing home safety and improving the homes of older people. Additional funding has been less important than new ways of working with existing resources, and basing professional workers locally has built up a closer and more knowledgeable relationship with service users and the area.

An important role for these additional resources is both to engage people already active in the community as service providers, organisers, campaigners or religious leaders, and to engage people who may not be involved in community activities or accessing services, and may be hard to reach. Substance misusers or people with mental health problems are examples. The challenge for a community development approach to engaging all sections of a local population is to link people in their neighbourhoods and communities with the wider planning structures where there is the power to shift resources or reshape how services are delivered. This is primarily about establishing influence with public bodies such as the local authority and the PCT, both through their own participation structures and the LSP. But it is also about linking up what is happening in the neighbourhood with other systems with which its residents interact, from schools to the health economy.

Neighbourhood Management initiatives have established local partnerships capable of improving communication between local residents and service providers, and giving residents more influence over local services (www.neighbourhoodmanagement.net). Local differences in health needs can be reflected in SLAs or charters agreed with neighbourhood partnerships that can be used to hold service users to account and judge success. Neighbourhood Management has the potential to take a holistic view of neighbourhood health needs and contribute to reducing health inequalities. It is a level at which neighbourhood teams of practitioners, and partnership boards with resident participation, can judge the suitability of services in meeting local needs and identify opportunities to improve coordination by co-locating services or referral from one service to another. While GPs may be regarded as the benchmark of community health provision in England, the experience of Neighbourhood Management initiatives to date has been that nurse- or health visitor-led services are more relevant to achieving change in the neighbourhood (Healthier Neighbourhoods Action Team, 2005).

The use of targets and performance management as devices to ensure delivery against political commitments made by government introduces a potential tension into neighbourhood-based work. When residents of a Neighbourhood Management pathfinder area in Rotherham were asked to define their own health indicators, it was not rates of heart disease or diabetes that figured but experiences such as 'feeling safe' and 'birds singing' (Healthier Neighbourhoods Action Team, 2005). Fewer boarded-up windows, being able to access affordable child care, and more outlets selling affordable healthy food were among the targets residents felt important to improving their health.

This can be resolved by nesting these local resident concerns within the 'official' targets as they are often underlying drivers. Neighbourhoods offer the means to connect everyday health concerns with the targets that frame national policies and commitments, and that enable comparisons to be made over time and across space as a way of auditing progress with implementation.

Neighbourhoods, however, are more than cases for the purpose of measuring gaps in floor targets, as if what matters are the health variables rather than the cases themselves. It is, as Ragin (2000) argues, the cases and their *states* that are important to a health strategy that factors in neighbourhoods because it is recognised that a rising tide of generally improving living standards will not lift all boats. In this book I have proposed that a useful, practical way of establishing what this state should be is to complement the 'decent homes' standard with a standard for 'decent neighbourhoods'. Some of the attributes of a decent neighbourhood can be derived from the evidence about health impacts reviewed in Chapter Four. Others need more research, such as the role of mixed-income communities in such a standard. Currently, it is an anomaly that in England we have an official definition of a 'decent home' and a rating system for assessing the health hazards that may exist inside a home, which can trigger intervention, but no equivalent for the residential environment beyond the front door.

Just as with decent homes, where we see housing falling in and out of the decency standard over time, neighbourhoods are dynamic. The system state of a neighbourhood depends on the state of order parameters such as the employment rate and interest rates. A neighbourhood with low housing demand may be a candidate for redevelopment to create a more 'sustainable' community at one time, but at another time a recovery of the wider housing market may increase demand, and fuel opposition to redevelopment among local residents. A decent neighbourhoods standard therefore needs to be adaptable and based on consultation, with neighbourhoods being able to opt out of some parts of the standard by agreement or enhance the standard, perhaps by paying a local Council Tax supplement. The way it triggers intervention should also be agreed with local residents. Otherwise, the standard would become another top–down target, with echoes of some of the insensitive redevelopment of the 1960s and 1970s. It was only a few decades ago that Newcastle City Council's chief planning officer felt able to write:

> One result of slum clearance is that a considerable movement of people takes place over long distances, with devastating effect on the social groupings built up over the years. However, one might argue that this is a good thing when we are dealing with people who have no initiative or civic pride. The task, surely, is to break up such groupings even though the people seem to be satisfied with their miserable environment.... (Burns, 1963, pp 93-4)

Although Burns was criticised for this attitude at the time, it was not an uncommon perspective among modernising bureaucrats in the 1960s. Indeed, Britain's post-war new towns strategy emphasised the 'balanced communities' of mixed occupations and social backgrounds they would create, contrasting these with the squalor of working-class slums in many of the old industrial areas. In 1946, the Labour government's planning minister stated in the House of Commons that, 'The aim must be to combine in the New Town the friendly spirit of the ... slum ... with the vastly improved health conditions of the new estate but it must be a broadened spirit embracing all classes of society' (cited in Robinson, 1983, p 268).

Recent studies have suggested that while housing renewal might have improved health conditions as an outcome when the process is over, the process itself can be health damaging. For some residents this may outweigh any health benefits (Allen, 2000; Ambrose, 2000). The impact of redevelopment and displacement on the lives of those affected should not be underestimated: it is a solution that needs to be applied in consultation with residents. Another issue with both HMR in England and HOPE VI in the US is that the most disadvantaged areas may be seen as having few prospects for attracting middle-income home buyers into redeveloped neighbourhoods. HOPE VI, for example, appears to have targeted not the most severely distressed public housing but sites that are most likely to attract higher-income development (National Housing Law Project et al, 2002). Not only may this mean a net loss of social housing in high-demand areas, but in areas of low demand the solution may simply become demolition and grassing over the resulting empty spaces, rather than any kind of revitalisation through redevelopment as a mixed community.

Perhaps the most troubling aspect of the 'mixed community' paradigm of current housing and planning policy is the patchy evidence base. While US studies in particular do point to overall health and other benefits arising from mixed-income rather than uniformly low-income neighbourhoods, there may be other less dramatic ways of achieving this benefit than redevelopment and displacement. Neighbourhood Management, for example, could achieve the collective efficacy thought to be more prevalent in middle-income areas. Similarly, a critical assessment of the HOPE VI programme by the National Housing Law Project et al (2002) found no evidence of building social capital in redeveloped areas, but did find that infrastructure and services improved. This was simply a result of the extra investment in child care and health care centres, job training programmes and retail space.

At the heart of this issue are the order parameters of any society, its phase space, and the extent of inequality these make possible. However much deprived neighbourhoods are renewed or replaced, if there is a wide scope for differences by income, wealth and neighbourhood in a society the deprived neighbourhood will reappear as where poor people live. So there is a need not to be too localist about this, and to view neighbourhoods in the bigger picture, not least because as open systems they are shaped by their environment and environmental inputs. Meeting the decent homes standard for English social housing, for example, has meant a huge input of resources on a national scale into neighbourhoods with some of the highest rates of deprivation in the country. Yet the sustainability of many of these neighbourhoods is still in doubt, with causes that lie substantially beyond localities in processes of spatial filtering driven by the wider income and wealth inequalities of a globalised economy.

From local to global: making connections and modelling the big picture

No analysis of social policy can ignore the impact of globalisation, and this is no less true of a study of neighbourhoods and health. Neighbourhood programmes are implemented in the context of a globalised economy and national welfare regimes that mediate, more or less strongly, between this economy and local lives. Can neighbourhoods be connected to this globalised world? What are the processes of globalisation that surround them?

Competition by low-wage countries with high-wage countries means that the latter are moving their production up the value chain through technological investment to compete as 'knowledge economies'. Because this increases demand and pay for highly skilled personnel, while reducing demand for less skilled workers, the process is often held responsible for the rising income inequality documented for most OECD countries during the 1980s and 1990s (Bjorvatn and Cappelen, 2004). Countries cannot respond, it is also often argued, by taxing highly paid personnel more heavily to narrow the widening pay gap because these personnel are internationally mobile and could relocate to where taxes are not being increased. Therefore, governments tend to settle for creating conditions that produce and attract knowledge workers, with their higher incomes boosting tax revenues even with tax cuts. The implications for income inequality are that it continues to grow unless measures are taken to equalise pre-tax incomes, one reason why some governments regard mass upskilling and higher education to be as much a social policy as an economic policy.

Democracies are unlikely to tolerate the extent of income inequality that globalisation will fuel without state intervention. Indeed, across the OECD as Gross Domestic Product (GDP) per capita has risen so has per capita social expenditure (OECD, 2005). Across the European

Union, the overall poverty rate of 15% would rise to 40% without income transfers through tax and spend cash benefits. There are, however, important differences between countries. The US may be richer than Sweden but the poor are much worse off. While Sweden's GDP per head is little more than two thirds that of the US, the poorest 20% of Swedish households are 40% better off than the poorest 20% of US households (Jackson and Segal, 2004). This is because income is more evenly distributed. Indeed, Kunst et al (2005) conclude from their survey of evidence about socioeconomic inequalities in health across 10 European states that, compared to other countries, the Nordic welfare states appear to have moderated the adverse effects of economic crises on the general health of disadvantaged sections of their populations. They also point out that the widening of inequalities in mortality seen in the UK during the 1980s was not as great as might be expected given the sharp rise in income inequality during this period. It seems likely that these effects will feed forward into future ill-health and may be a reason why inequalities in life expectancy are continuing to widen despite mild but progressively redistributive policy measures since 1997 (Shaw, 2005). The fact that redistribution has occurred at all in the UK is significant, given that it has been difficult to tackle relative deprivation when average incomes have been rising appreciably.

The world's developed welfare states may find it increasingly difficult to win public support for levels of redistributive taxation that keep up with the continuing pulling away of high earners in the income distribution (Bjorvatn and Cappelen, 2004). It seems likely that the growing income inequality evident in many OECD countries during the 1980s and 1990s will intensify, although it is difficult to pin this on globalisation alone because of the influence of other factors such as technological development (Brune and Garrett, 2005). Nevertheless, there are potent mixes of factors building up for developed welfare states. To the dynamic of widening income distributions, for example, can be added the economic pressures of ageing populations and declining fertility.

Economic growth is widely seen as a way out of these pressures, although with a neo-liberal drift towards privatisation and more conditionality in the provision of welfare services and benefits. There is little doubt that many less developed countries need growth, but in developed countries there are already arguments being made that further growth in GDP per head is unlikely to add to such a basic human aspiration as happiness. It may actually undermine the security of income and work, and the quality and stability of family and friendship relationships, that human beings need most to be happy (Layard, 2005). Growth could also be destroying the natural resources and systems on which any economic activity and human life depend, unless huge strides are made to achieve environmentally sustainable development (Hamilton, 2003).

A further problem is that economic growth is not even. We have to move up a level to the regional scale to see this clearly in the UK, and in many ways the increasing focus on smaller and smaller scales of deprivation clouds our view. Super Output Areas (SOAs) have been introduced to enable deprivation to be identified at a very small scale of localities of around 1,500 people. Moving back up a few levels of administrative geography reveals stark patterns by English region. The North East of England, for example, has over a fifth of its SOAs in the 10% of most deprived SOAs in England and over half in the 30% of most deprived. Only 35 are in the least deprived 10%. By contrast, the South East of England has little over 1% of its SOAs in the 10% most deprived in the country, and a quarter in the 10% least deprived. Almost all of the urban areas of the North East are either deprived or adjacent to a deprived area, while the opposite is the case in the South East. The underlying cause of this divided geography is the different positions of the two regions in the international division of labour, with economic globalisation having transformed the North East from an industrial heartland to a post-industrial hinterland, while the South East benefits from London's world city status as a financial and business services centre in the global economy. While the North East has lost large numbers of skilled industrial jobs and gained some new but routine service jobs, the South East has gained large numbers of higher-paid services jobs. Government policy has sought to protect the position of the London economy, given its contribution to the UK's global trading position, but at a cost to manufacturing jobs in the North East, which continue to move abroad.

A problem for post-industrial consumer societies is how to see and act on these bigger pictures when individualisation and disillusionment with politics are so widespread. The neighbourhood can be brought back in for this purpose, connecting the visible and close encounter we have with this small system to the wider systems with which it interacts. Cilliers (1998) describes this as the complexity concept of 'distributed representation', whereby patterns that have causal implications at a local scale – that are experienced in our neighbourhoods – only become clear by moving up a scale. A deprived neighbourhood, for instance, only makes sense as a concept in terms of contrasts with other neighbourhoods. This partitioning of space, and the sorting of people in space, are encoded in higher-level systems that generate these spatial inequalities downstream. The coordinates of a phase space captures this idea, defining the range of possible locations for a neighbourhood along variables that define neighbourhood attributes and combine with causal effects in particular places. This range may be very wide in some countries but quite narrow in others.

The opposite is also true: there is a feed-forward from neighbourhoods to larger systems. What we do locally may produce something globally that our local actions did not intend. Complexity theory is about trying to understand how this happens. The connection between local and global may have been apparent when the global for most people meant the boundaries of a single settlement or small region, but it is now far harder to 'see' what is happening up a few scales from our local experience. We tend to perceive events as different things happening in different places rather than as emerging wholes. Global warming is perhaps the exception but social emergence is getting less attention.

Until recently there has been no macroscope for seeing these societal wholes in dynamic and interactive ways, but computers and the worldwide web are changing this. Pioneering in this respect has been a team at the University of British Columbia in Vancouver, which has developed a computer game for residents living in the Georgia Basin to explore policy options for their region. Called QUEST and inspired by the videogame SimCity, it aims to help the public to understand alternative futures for complex and interacting ecological, social and economic systems (see www.basinfutures.net). The game enables players to generate scenarios for the region based on options chosen from a menu of goals. These could be full employment, more land set aside for parks, lower housing densities, or less deaths from vehicle accidents. The computer works with the player's chosen options and shows how they interact, conflict, or reinforce each other when the scenario is run forward. The idea behind QUEST is to demonstrate the emergent, system-wide consequences of individual decisions, particularly the consequences for the sustainability of the system. The game's designers do not see the main challenge for sustainable development to be a lack of policy or technical tools. Instead, they see the challenge to be a lack of public understanding of how individual choices about single issues interrelate to produce surprising collective outcomes, including undesired outcomes that, if known, would alter the choice made in the first place.

A further example of how modelling can be used to explore a type of emergence is the work of Mitchell et al (2000) that simulated what geographical patterns in Britain's health would look like under different national policy scenarios. They modelled the effects of changes in *national* levels of income inequality, unemployment and childhood poverty on *local* health outcomes for each of Britain's 723 parliamentary constituencies. The model assumes that the statistical relationship between income inequality and premature mortality is causal. So if tax changes were used to take income inequality from its level in the early 1990s back to the lower level of the early 1980s, an estimated 7,500 premature deaths each year could be prevented. Their modelling suggests that further lives could be saved by eliminating unemployment and eradicating childhood poverty. They also found some anomalous constituencies where deaths were either higher or lower than would be expected from the statistical relationships using national data, but these area effects were very much exceptions.

The message of Mitchell et al's work is that the outputs of national macroeconomic and social policies are order parameters that structure local outcomes. The implication is that ABIs are likely to have little impact by comparison. Their modelling, however, rather underplays local geography, both because parliamentary constituencies are a relatively large spatial scale at which to consider area effects, and because geography itself is likely to be a barrier to national programmes turning around conditions in the worst neighbourhoods. As argued in earlier chapters, linear statistical models measuring independent effects are not a good fit with social reality, especially when non-linear change and interaction are likely. The interaction of national policy measures with small areas will have non-linear and emergent effects.

This is not to deny the force of Mitchell et al's message. The persistence of problems such as health inequalities and deprived neighbourhoods continues to demand a macroperspective. Order parameters have a determining potential, but they may not determine outcomes if local conditions present a barrier. Similarly, local conditions have a causal potential but may not achieve this unless the state of order parameters is conducive to them having this effect. The order parameter of the general level of employment, for example, makes a large difference as to whether individual attributes of education, ethnicity, age or interview technique predict a person's risk of unemployment (Davey-Smith et al, 2001). Adjust this parameter value and the behaviour of individuals and the barriers and opportunities they face appear quite different.

Even in low unemployment societies problems of poverty and inequality persist. Mackenbach and Bakker (2002) show that in the

Nordic countries of Europe, with their long histories of relatively egalitarian social and economic policies, inequalities in self-reported morbidity are still substantial. These are being accentuated by the general trend towards better health status being more marked among higher-income groups. Although these countries continue to comprise a distinctive social-democratic welfare regime, typified by high rates of female employment, a more equal distribution of incomes, and more universal provision of public services across all social classes, they have not eliminated social exclusion. The extremes of the US's racialised urban ghettos and gated communities, or even the UK's inner-city deprivation and outer 'sink' estates, are absent. But those at the bottom of the income and education scales still live more segregated lives in the most deprived housing areas, often ethnically concentrated.

The concept of social exclusion recognises how exclusion from what others take for granted can result not just from income inequality but also from differences of age, gender, geographical location and ethnicity. These are attributes that often interact together and cluster with wider parameters such as the unemployment level to create concentrated disadvantage. There is, however, human agency at work in these processes, even if this is agency that has emergent, unintended effects. Social exclusion is more than a phenomenon that just happens to some people; it is done to some people by other people, whether wittingly or not. By paying high prices for homes in decent neighbourhoods others are excluded from them, by commuting long distances to jobs others who live nearby are denied them, and by taking the car to shop in a supermarket others who cannot drive are denied its choice and prices as their local shops close down.

There is no escaping the role of values in the triad of evidence, resources and values that combine to produce policy and practice decisions. How far are the UK's current strategies to renew neighbourhoods and reduce health inequalities value-based? Wicked issues such as neighbourhood deprivation and health inequalities have become significant because they drive up public spending and are perceived as risks to many more people than just those directly affected (Beck, 1992; Moran, 2001). Are these strategies, then, aiming to do just enough to contain costs to taxpayers and protect their health, or are they aiming at a qualitative transformation, an epidemiological transition, in the health of people living in poor places? In the case of health inequalities, the spending and economic implications of not taking action are prominent in policy discourse (Wanless, 2002, 2004; HM Treasury, 2004, 2005). This may make us cynical about the intent of governments claiming to have strategies that will achieve a real difference to inequality, but there is also a moral imperative for individuals. We all create distinctions between ourselves and others through everyday actions such as choosing or avoiding particular jobs, places to live, schools for our children and consumer lifestyles. The wider the space of possibilities in these respects, the more discriminating we are likely to be and the more unequal society is likely to become. This is where the fundamental debate lies: the boundaries, limits and relativities we think are reasonable for our society. At what levels of income and wealth should progressive taxation start to narrow what the market would otherwise continue to widen? At what levels of segregation by class or ethnicity should governments intervene with planning and housing measures to desegregate what markets would continue to segregate? What should be the target per cent reduction in cancer mortality between the worst 20% of local authority areas and the national average?

It is easier for policy to determine minimum standards of income or housing conditions than to intervene in these relativities. Some ways of intervening are more direct than others. Income inequality can be very directly addressed with taxation, but also indirectly addressed by narrowing the inequalities that drive differences in income such as in education and skills. A decent neighbourhoods standard may help to stem the selective out-migration of people and capital that creates neighbourhood 'concentration effects' because intervention would be triggered by falling below the standard. But people cannot be prevented from moving from less desirable to more desirable neighbourhoods, even if the emergent effect of these movements is to create much wider divides than individuals would actually choose themselves. And markets will continue to offer this choice and stimulate upmarket moves if there is no ceiling on just how decent a neighbourhood can be.

This is why floor targets are so important. They track inequalities in the key dimensions of welfare that people are most concerned about, and they drive programmes of intervention. Many neighbourhoods in the 1980s and 1990s were left to cope with poverty and a rise in crime, drugs, antisocial behaviour, dereliction, failing services, stigma and ill-health, often already having suffered brutalist redevelopment in the 1960s and 1970s. Various ABIs were aimed at these problems, but none were framed within a national policy system focused on narrowing gaps. The programmes were also short term and had little long-term effect. They were frequently undermined by the open system nature of neighbourhoods as residents either moved out or became trapped in workless ghettos where, if new jobs did arrive, they could be taken by commuters, in-migrants or new labour market entrants.

The current NR and health inequality strategies do not have all the answers and progress is slow. Weak demand for labour and mismatches between skills and demand remain very difficult to solve. But there is little doubt that a big push is under way to turn around the poor liveability of the most deprived neighbourhoods and strengthen the focus of the NHS on the health of their residents. The performance management regimes that encompass the NHS, local government and LSPs are being focused on wicked issues, and are keeping on the agenda of these organisations the aim of closing gaps. The weaknesses of these regimes, principally the lack of connection between evidence-informed processes and how they will meet targets, are as much a reflection of the failure of social policy research to keep up with these developments as defects of the regimes themselves.

What the research evidence does make clear is that the English NR strategy is likely to make only a small contribution to tackling health inequality, given that the wider determinants of health lie beyond the neighbourhood system. But it is making a difference and could make more of a difference with a stronger focus on the attributes reviewed in Chapter Four. Of more significance in the long term, and the reason why this book has devoted so many pages to it, is the performance management infrastructure and the way it makes transparent what is happening between places and between people. The joined-up performance management regime, which is now emerging as an audit of places as well as organisations, means that the issue of gaps between unhealthy places and national averages *counts* on the agendas of chief executives and politicians running the mainstream budgets and services that dwarf the budget for the NR strategy. Particularly crucial in this respect is how the health of residents can be improved faster in the most deprived locales. National targets are necessary in this context because they enable comparison. In terms of inequality they may be incremental rather than transformative. But if, as targets are reached, they become milestones on the way to new targets in the same direction of travel, then this incremental change could, in time, amount to a transformation. ABIs have been criticised for not being 'structural' interventions, but this is fundamentally an issue of them needing to endure long enough to engender structural change. Structure is enduring agency. The initiatives may be seen as slow in achieving this, but this is largely due to the lack of public pressure to see rapid change in an indicator such as a health floor target compared to a hospital waiting list.

New ways of working

As well as the importance of floor targets as a type of macroscope, the NR and health inequality strategies being pursued in the UK are important in stimulating new ways of working and structural change in governance arrangements. Globalisation is a driver of change in how public policy is delivered, because of pressure both to achieve competitive advantage in a global economy and to open up services to international competition. The search for both efficiency and effectiveness from public services includes more closely matching services to needs, achieving better integration across services, and making much more use of research evidence about 'what works' (Walter et al, 2005; Wimbush et al, 2005; www.publichealth.nice.org.uk). In many countries, greater use is being made of the private sector as a source of investment through public–private partnerships, of spare capacity to deal with demand pressures, of management expertise, and of alternative provision. Overlaying all this is a strengthening of performance management as public bodies acquire a planning and commissioning role in relation to a more diverse range of providers of service. While these developments are often criticised as a neo-liberal turn in the policies of even left-of-centre governments, there is no necessary connection between globalisation and a dismantling of welfare states. It has already been noted that across the OECD as GDP per capita has risen so has per capita social expenditure, but it is the differences between countries that are of more note than any general trend across all countries. Social expenditure as a percentage of GDP reaches 25%-30% among the developed welfare states of countries such as Sweden, France and Italy, compared to less than 20% in Australia, Japan or Ireland, despite very similar GDPs per capita (OECD, 2005). In general, national welfare regimes are pretty much 'locked in' by the norms and institutions of their societies. But the complexity of their societies is growing and public services reform is responding, although within the parameters of different welfare regimes.

Across taxation and social spending there is little evidence that the capacity of states to self-organise in these spheres has been reduced by economic globalisation. Domestic factors remain significant in how taxation is distributed. The strength of organised labour and its political power are still important in influencing where the tax burden falls (Weiss, 2003; Ellison, 2005). There have been cuts in benefits and eligibility, cost controls and privatisations, but these have sat alongside expansions of other social programmes, with benefits and entitlements becoming more generous in some areas. The Wanless reports on the

NHS, for example, emphasised the importance of spending more on public health interventions, particularly among the most disadvantaged groups, as a way of reducing pressures on treatment services. While Wanless supported the UK government's substantial real increases in NHS funding, he emphasised the need for upstream measures to manage the growing demand for health care downstream (Wanless, 2004).

Wanless' preventative approach led him to identify important gaps in the public health evidence base, especially studies of the relative effectiveness of different interventions and their economic evaluation. 'Preventative' measures, for instance, may actually increase spending downstream. Sure Start has increased health and social services use among families in the targeted areas and increased the number of children identified as having Special Educational Needs and therefore entitled to additional service inputs (Barnes, J. et al, 2005). Adults receiving means-tested Income Support have also increased, although the unemployment rate has fallen more in Sure Start areas than the decline nationally. Other services that show a rise in use should save expenditure downstream, such as immunisations, and clearly all the Sure Start programmes are premised on the notion of investment early in children's lives that can prevent more costly interventions in youth or adulthood (in this respect, some of the Sure Start national evaluation findings are worrying. Compared to England averages, birth weight has dropped significantly in Sure Start areas and neonatal and infant mortality has risen. There is evidence that services such as child health clinics are not reaching the most vulnerable women).

While there remains significant policy space for governments to develop programmes according to domestic rather than global imperatives, globalisation does frame what governments can do. Weiss (2003) argues that the vulnerabilities of nation states in the global economy do present their governments with new challenges. How they respond, however, is influenced by national norms – social partnership in Sweden, economic nationalism in Japan, Korea or Taiwan, and the state intervention of French *étatisme* for example. She also suggests that global economic interdependence is transforming how governments act. In particular, governments are managing specific areas of major risk by partnering with domestic business and labour organisations, as well as with international bodies, to arrive at joint approaches to these risks. Governments set the goals in this scenario but their transformational capacity operates through these alliances and networks.

There is, according to Wright's (2000) analysis, a spreading and deepening complexity in the world as a result of globalisation and the cumulative effects of what he calls win–win gaming. In the policy field, win–win gaming is about finding collaborative advantages within a shared space or 'whole system', which for an LSP or LAA is the local authority area. This is the system where 'theories of change' link activity and outcomes in a 'post-bureaucratic' social policy working in a zone of complexity where certainty and agreement about how activities relate to outcomes are issues for investigation and experimentation.

LSPs are above all an attempt to work on a whole-system basis across all public services rather than just those, such as health and social care, where there are obvious pathways that cut across organisational boundaries. The 'ideal type' for an LSP is a complex adaptive system comprising agents whose actions are interconnected and who can learn. There is, therefore, a need for LSPs to be strongly oriented to using evidence within their performance management frameworks, with their programmes having the status of a set of propositions about theories of change.

For the evidence-informed practice paradigm to work there need to be conditions for learning to take place. Unfortunately there are often not the resources or time for this to happen (Coote et al, 2004). Atkinson et al's (2006) review of urban policies and health in the UK found that there has been little systematic storage and cataloguing of either programme documentation or evaluations. This is changing with the development of websites for storing and disseminating this type of material, such as the NRU's (www.renewal.net) website. However, evidence-based policy and practice is not a linear process of producing knowledge and then applying it. Even the theory of change approach, which engages the researcher and the practitioner in co-theorising and co-inquiry, has been criticised for failing to recognise the reality of multiple discourses surrounding issues, the shifts in priorities that occur during programmes, the power of local context to modify programmes and their results, or the unintended consequences that fall outside the ambit of predetermined measures of effectiveness (Barnes et al, 2003). Nevertheless, the theory of change approach introduces an important discipline into policy implementation. It enables a model to be set up: a simulation that clarifies supposed causal relationships and interdependencies, with a view to learning from feedback and adapting so that implementation closes in on the outcome (Fitz-Gibbon, 1996; Gilbert and Troitzsch, 1999).

The aim, as Ragin (2000, p 203) puts it, is 'The identification of manipulable necessary conditions' to achieve an outcome. Ragin also identifies why achieving change in complex zones like health inequalities is so difficult compared to just health improvement. Banning smoking in public spaces is likely to improve general health, but we can be far less certain about whether it will narrow health inequalities because achieving a faster cessation rate among the groups with the highest levels of smoking is an issue of *enablement* rather than *constraint*. Ragin (2000, pp 203-4) writes:

> It is important to point out that while necessary conditions may both constrain and enable outcomes, enablement is much more difficult to achieve than constraint. To set the stage for an outcome – to create a situation where it can occur – all the necessary conditions for that outcome must be in place. To prevent an outcome, by contrast, all that is required is to remove or interfere with a single necessary condition. It is clear that enablement requires a much greater depth of knowledge about social life than constraint. To focus on necessary conditions, especially with prevention in mind, is to highlight the fragility of social accomplishment and the ubiquity of disruption.

Enabling transformational outcomes

How realistic is it to see the NR strategy as having transformational capacity, achieving a 'phase transition' from an unhealthy to a healthy attractor for its targeted neighbourhoods? The challenge is enormous in those areas where problems have become deeply entrenched. For example, in the 2% of most deprived neighbourhoods in England the rate of worklessness is 50% higher than in the next 8% of neighbourhoods, and more than three-and-a-half times the national average (Berube, 2005). Incremental improvements are unlikely to deliver any breakthrough in the face of such concentrated problems.

Worklessness is the biggest barrier to creating a situation where NR can occur and is a very significant driver of ill-health. Many old industrial areas have relatively low rates of economic activity among their working-age populations. This is partly associated with people leaving the workforce on grounds of ill-health arising from working in industries such as coal mining. But a recent pattern has emerged of high inactivity rates combining with high unemployment rates. This suggests that much unemployment in these areas is disguised. A 'discouraged worker' phenomenon arises whereby employers are reluctant to hire people with a sickness record or whose age is regarded as a risk, and people still of working age have little incentive to find employment if local jobs pay little more than their income from disability or sickness benefits, and may be considerably less secure. The increase and persistence in levels of economic inactivity due to sickness and disability is one of the main challenges facing area-based programmes in the UK.

Among new measures to support people who have been ill or are disabled back into employment is an emphasis on GPs and the NHS helping to overcome barriers to employment rather than simply assessing patients as unfit to work. Work advisors are being located in some GP surgeries along with advice on in-work benefits. Pilots to test this approach are being rolled out, along with benefit changes designed to reward claimants who seek work, and provide better incomes for those too severely sick or disabled to take up any employment (the Pathways to Work programme, see www.dwp.gov.uk). The spatial concentration of worklessness is being targeted by the 'Working Neighbourhoods Pilot', which focuses additional support with overcoming barriers to employment on neighbourhoods with very high numbers of Incapacity Benefit claimants (www.jobcentreplus.gov.uk). The prevention of health-related worklessness is a focus of programmes to reduce illness or accidents caused at work and to improve rehabilitation, from national health and safety legislation and guidance to improving occupational health services (www.hse.gov.uk).

The NHS itself has an important role as a major employer and developer able to provide job opportunities directly or through procurement of goods and services and local building and refurbishment programmes. Some existing hospitals have adopted this agenda, especially those located near areas of deprivation where tailored training and employment schemes can contribute both to improving health and recruiting and retaining trained employees. In the English West Midlands the SHA launched an award-winning scheme in 2003 with seven local NHS organisations including University Hospital Birmingham, one of the biggest hospitals in the NHS (Shannon, 2005). Assisting Communities to Identify Vocational Areas of Training and Employment (ACTIVATE) has targeted reducing worklessness among long-term unemployed people, BME groups, refugees, single parents and people with drug or alcohol problems. The initiative provides job-readiness training, work experience and mentoring. The first phase of the scheme funded by £1.7 million from the European Social Fund saw 453 people complete over two years; 182 found a job and 25% took up further training. Forty per cent of people entering the scheme were from BME communities and the second phase plans to increase this to 65%.

There are similar vocational rehabilitation programmes elsewhere, often basing employment advisors and occupational therapists with clinical teams and providing ongoing support through care plans. In London, the South West London and St George's Mental Health NHS Trust integrated an employment specialist with the Early Intervention Service for young people with first-episode psychosis, achieving after one year an increase in the employment rate from 10% to 40% and a decline in the proportion not engaged in employment, education or training from 55% to 5% (NRU, 2005b). Thus, the NHS can contribute to health improvement not just as a service provider but also as an agent of regeneration. It is a major employer, landowner and purchaser of goods and services. It also has a substantial impact on the environment, consuming energy and generating travel. A recent report from the King's Fund noted a commitment from the UK government to promoting health and sustainable development, but argued that the two agendas were not well connected (Coote, 2002). The considerable potential of the NHS to achieve health and sustainability dividends from its spending was being impeded by performance being measured on other criteria, notably financial and clinical targets.

Targets incentivise performance, but neither targets nor the programmes designed to deliver them achieve change on their own. Pawson (2002) points out that it is the reasons or resources that programmes provide which engender change. Nicotine replacement therapy will not achieve smoking cessation unless smokers have a reason to quit. Nicotine replacement therapy is a resource that will work for many people motivated to quit but not if there are reasons to continue smoking. If neighbourhoods that were regarded as unsafe are made safer, people who smoke have more of a reason to give up. If a neighbourhood is improved with more greenery, better paths, cleaner streets and convenient local shops, residents may have reasons to take exercise locally and walk more often which they did not have before. If resources are spent on improved housing, better local job prospects and more accessible primary health care, then health is likely to improve for the people who benefit from these resources.

Pawson's argument is a 'realist synthesis', based on realist social theory and its conceptualisation of phenomena as context-contingent outcomes of underlying generative mechanisms. Thus, the mechanisms or *drivers* that give interventions their efficacy are the resources and reasons that they mobilise, but this efficacy also depends on contextual conditions. These include the attributes of the people meant to benefit and the circumstances of implementation. For example, it may only be older women who walk more if neighbourhoods offer convenient destinations, an effect that may be missed by a general sample survey (King et al, 2003). Or the potential health benefits of housing improvements may be undermined by the disruption and uncertainty caused by the way the improvements programme is managed, or the impact of subsequent rent increases on the ability of low-income tenants to buy nutritious and healthy food. Interventions have an *outcome pattern* rather than a single effect, so that evaluations of their impact need to consider the range of effects, which may include unintended consequences.

As Pawson also points out, learning from 'what works' should not be about transferring programmes from where they worked to where they might work again, but about testing a *theory of change* in a new context. The theory may work in some contexts but not in others. So, evaluation needs to be concerned not with whether an intervention simply works or does not work, but with receptive and non-receptive contexts (with the need to do something else in the case of the latter). For example, an improved neighbourhood or someone finding work, like a supportive household context, is likely not only to help promote giving up smoking, but also to create a receptive context for smoking cessation interventions such as free nicotine replacement therapy.

There are three reasons why an intervention may not work. It may not be the right thing to do; it may be the right thing but done in the wrong way; or it may be undermined by its context and contextual factors working against it. Frequently the problem is one of resources and not enough resource 'energy' being put into a system to achieve a phase transition rather than small, incremental change. There are two answers to this: spend more on interventions that are likely to work so that they have a bigger effect, or manage existing resources to achieve a bigger impact. In general, it is worth looking at whether the most is being achieved from existing resources before putting in more resources. This is where an initiative such as LAAs is important. LAAs, if they work properly, are about better targeting, removing duplication, achieving critical mass and finding non-zero-sum solutions.

Non-zero-sumness

I have decided to finish this book with an affirmation of Wright's (2000) optimistic account of how the world's societies are travelling along a trajectory of growing complexity in which globalisation is the latest stage. I have already connected the projects of recent innovations such as LSPs and LAAs with imperatives arising from globalisation, and in the governance field they seem to me to fit with Wright's argument that there is in biological, cultural and, I would add, policy evolution a thread of 'long-run growth in non-zero-sumness' (Wright, 2000, p 243). This is a dynamic of mutually beneficial, self-interested cooperation traceable through history, despite the many counter-examples, but remarkable for the way it appears to be built into the fabric of things and give change a directionality.

In the short run, when agents are in interaction with each other a variety of outcomes is possible, but in the long run these interactions produce, more often than not, outcomes that are positive sums for the parties involved. This dynamic has driven the planet's organisms to higher levels of complexity, out of which arose human intelligence and consciousness. Individual units, whether cells, animals or communities, cooperate in ways that achieve a net benefit for all, and these win-win interactions are driven forward by evolution exploiting and selecting for them. Now cultural evolution continues with the same underlying directionality and growing social complexity. Over more than 300 pages, Wright presents his evidence for this thesis, primarily by considering the cultural evolution of humans from hunter-gatherer societies to the emergence of nation states and now globalisation.

An awareness of shared space is a key driver of non-zero-sum gaming. It could explain both the emergence of neighbourhoods as 'communities' and their relative decline as shared spaces of communication and trust. In increasingly complex societies neighbourhoods coexist with wider and deeper types of collective consciousness, such as diaspora or virtual communities. But their particular importance as residential space means that neighbourhoods continue to have social and political significance. If one definition of a system is a bundle of information processing, storage and analysis that leads to adaptive collective behaviours, then neighbourhoods are systems despite the growing complexity around them (Dembski, 2003). Information gets shared in neighbourhoods, passively and actively, but among many more sources of information than have existed in the past. In particular, there is more comparative information, which informs how people feel about their neighbourhoods. Signs of decline and further deterioration to come, communicated by 'broken windows', are sufficient to prompt moving out of a neighbourhood for those who can and to depress the health of people who remain in conditions that they know are better elsewhere. Large differences in health and neighbourhood conditions create zero-sum situations, such as a reluctance of the healthy to pay for health care for the unhealthy, and withdrawal into segregated, even gated, communities.

Wright's argument is that there is an underlying tendency for non-zero-sum solutions to emerge even when relationships have been overwhelmingly zero-sum. This occurs as previously hostile or competing interests realise that there is a scale at which problems can have non-zero-sum solutions. This is the significance of the QUEST project: using information technology as a macroscope for non-zero-sumness on the basis that at a regional, national and global scale people are in the same boat. The NR strategy's performance management system is also an example, tracking gaps in conditions between the 'worst' areas and England as a whole, and making this information publicly accessible. Even with neighbourhood internet sites, as access to the web widens, more and more people will have the opportunity to reconnoitre a neighbourhood remotely – a democratisation of knowledge previously largely confined to those with the resources and networks to do such things. This information could fuel demands that something is done about neighbourhoods that score poorly, in the same way that attention is focused on schools and hospitals that score poorly in their performance assessments.

Wright's analysis is that information is one of two critical conditions for non-zero-sumness to emerge: the other is trust. If neighbourhood profiles on the internet are going to drive deepening neighbourhood social divisions, it is because people are likely to move to areas where there are others they can trust – who are like them. This, Wright argues, is a type of extension of altruism among kin to a reciprocal altruism among wider groups of people that has formed the basis of social organisation. Reciprocal altruism is social capital, a form of alliance and source of social support, expressed as a moral code and policed by behaviours such as tit-for-tat. This is not because altruism is good in a purely moral sense, but because it creates the basis for trust as a way of surviving among finite resources, being healthy and happy. Failing in this respect is a route to disease and premature death. Alongside social capital, however, is status-seeking, the reason why competition and cooperation coexist. Marmot's (2004) work has already been reviewed about the dangers of the 'status syndrome' for our health, but status-seeking will not go away. Status, Wright argues, is largely ascribed to people who deliver a benefit to others: we raise our standing by impressing others. At its best this drives progress and improvement, while at its worst it introduces damaging gulfs between us as our own position becomes experienced as subordination rather than status.

Wright's focus on non-zero-sumness as a strategy adopted throughout biological and cultural evolution finds its echo in social policy and the contemporary emphasis on partnership working and shared priorities. What works is frequently what delivers win-win outcomes. The concern of regional and local strategic partnerships with 'closing gaps' is not just an issue of social justice but of economic efficiency and containing public spending, as the Wanless (2002, 2004) reports so clearly argued in relation to health inequalities and their impact on NHS expenditure. Tackling health inequality for Wanless is a win-win strategy. The current emphasis on learning, and on knowledge-based or evidence-informed practice, is also a reflection of Wright's argument that as complexity grows, intelligence increases. There are even signs of a further elaboration of complexity here with a democratisation of the use of information and evidence, and an expectation that users and the public are stakeholders in research and performance assessment ('nothing about us without us'). New types of engagement and involvement are emerging from this, throwing up new issues and more complexity.

The neighbourhood, amid this growing complexity, has some stability associated with its status as home ground. People generally care about where they live and about human potential being wasted when lives are cut short prematurely. These two agendas of caring for places and realising everyone's full potential are important justifications for state intervention in neighbourhoods and the determinants of health. They connect what people are concerned about locally with the big picture of the nature of society. This book has argued that recent policy developments in England have put in place frameworks for this intervention on a societal scale, drawing upon performance management as a tool of social policy and moving it into the uncharted waters of wicked issues and whole systems. There is still a lot to do, both to improve how local practice can be modelled more plausibly to connect with targets and their trajectories, and to marry the bottom-up agenda of neighbourhood participation and governance with national floor targets. The success of this work should be reflected in the progress made with reducing inequalities in health. This progress depends above all, however, on looking beyond concerns with just neighbourhood liveability and health care to society and its governance, which still largely shape the space of possibilities for decent neighbourhoods and health.

References

Abbott, R. D., White, L. R., Ross, G. W., Masaki, K. H., Curb, J. D. and Petrovitch, H. (2004) 'Walking and dementia in physically capable elderly men', *Journal of the American Medical Association*, 292 (12), pp 1447-53.

Acheson, D. (Chair) (1998) *Independent Inquiry into Inequalities in Health Report*, London: The Stationery Office.

Adams, J. and White, M. (2005) 'Socio-economic deprivation is associated with increased proximity to general practices in England: an ecological analysis', *Journal of Public Health*, 27, pp 80-1.

Alexander, L. M., Inchley, J., Todd, J., Currie, D., Cooper, A. R. and Currie, C. (2005) 'The broader impact of walking to school among adolescents: seven day accelerometry based study', *British Medical Journal*, 331, pp 1061-2.

Allen, T. (2000) 'Housing renewal – doesn't it make you sick?', *Housing Studies*, 15 (3), pp 443-61.

Almedom, A. M. (2005) 'Social capital and mental health: an interdisciplinary review of primary evidence', *Social Science & Medicine*, 61, pp 943-64.

Alvarez-Rosete, A., Bevan, G., Mays, N. and Dixon, J. (2005) 'Effect of diverging policy across the NHS', *British Medical Journal*, 331, pp 946-50.

Ambrose, P. (2000) *A Drop in the Ocean: The health Gain from the Central Stepney SRB in the Context of National Health Inequalities*, Brighton: The Health and Social Policy Research Centre, University of Brighton.

Ambrose, P., Barlow, J., Bonsey, A., Pullin, M., Donkin, V. and Randles, J. (1996) *The Real Cost of Poor Homes*, London: The Royal Institution of Chartered Surveyors.

Amin, A. (2002) 'Spatialities of globalisation', *Environment and Planning A*, 34 (3), pp 385-99.

Anderson, L. (2005) 'Using Data to Support Evidence-Based Corporate Strategy: A Case Study of Middlesbrough Council', Unpublished M.Prof thesis, University of Teesside.

Archer, M. (1995) *Realist Social Theory: The Morphogenetic Approach*, Cambridge, England: Cambridge University Press.

Ardern, K. (2004) 'HIA: a practitioner's view', in J. Kemm, J. Parry and S. Palmer (eds) *Health Impact Assessment*, Oxford: Oxford University Press, pp 103-14.

Ashton, J. and Seymour, H. (1988) *The New Public Health*, Milton Keynes: Open University Press.

Asthana, S. and Halliday, J. (2006) *What Works In Tackling Health Inequalities?*, Bristol: The Policy Press.

Atkinson, R., Thomson, H., Kearns, A. and Petticrew, M. (2006) 'Giving urban policy its 'medical': assessing the place of health in area-based regeneration', *Policy & Politics*, 34 (1), pp 5–26.

Audit Commission (2003) *Achieving the NHS Plan: Assessment of Current Performance, Likely Future Progress and Capacity to Improve*, London: Audit Commission.

Audit Scotland (2006) *Overview of the Local Authority Audits 2005*, Edinburgh: Audit Scotland.

Auditor General for Wales (2006) *Wales Programme for Improvement Annual Report 2004/2005*, Cardiff: Wales Audit Office.

Babb, P., Martin, J. and Haezewindt, P. (2004) *Focus on Social Inequalities*, London: HMSO.

Balfour, J. L. and Kaplan, G. A. (2002) 'Neighborhoood environment and loss of physical function in older adults: evidence from the Alameda County Study', *American Journal of Epidemiology*, 155, pp 507–15.

Ball, M. and Maginn, P. J. (2004) 'The contradictions of urban policy: the case of the Single Regeneration Budget in London', *Environment and Planning C*, 22, pp 739–65.

Barnes, J., Desousa, C., Frost, M., Harper, G. and Laban, D. (2005) *National Evaluation Report: Changes in the Characteristics of Sure Start Local Programmes Areas in Rounds 1 to 4 between 2000/2001 and 2002/2003*, London: HMSO.

Barnes, M., Matka, E. and Sullivan, H. (2003) 'Evidence, understanding and complexity', *Evaluation*, 9 (3), pp 265–84.

Barnes, M., Bauld, L., Benzeval, M., Judge, K., Mackenzie, M. and Sullivan, H. (2005) *Health Action Zones: Partnerships for Health Equity*, London: Routledge.

Barrow, M. and Bachan, R. (1997) *The Real Cost of Poor Homes: Footing the Bill*, London: The Royal Institution of Chartered Surveyors.

Bartley, M. (2004) *Health Inequality*, Cambridge: Polity.

Bate, R., Best, R. and Holmans, A. (eds) (2000) *On the Move: The Housing Consequences of Migration*, York: York Publishing Services.

Battersby, S., Landon, M., Moore, R., Ormandy, D. and Wilkinson, P. (2002) *Statistical Evidence to Support the Housing, Health and Safety Rating System*, Vols 1–3, London: ODPM.

Batty, M. (2005) *Cities and Complexity*, London: The MIT Press.

Bauld, L., Judge, K., Barnes, M., Benzeval, M., MacKenzie, M. and Sullivan, H. (2005) 'Promoting social change: the experience of Health Action Zones in England', *Journal of Social Policy*, 43 (3), pp 427-45.

Beck, U. (1992) *Risk Society: Towards a New Modernity*, London: Sage Publications.

Benzeval, M. (2005) 'Tackling health inequalities', in M. Barnes, L. Bauld, M. Benzeval, K. Judge, M. Mackenzie and H. Sullivan (2005) *Health Action Zones: Partnerships for Health Equity*, London: Routledge, pp 138-56.

Berube, A. (2005) *Mixed Communities in England: A US Perspective on Evidence and Policy Prospects*, York: Joseph Rowntree Foundation.

Bevan, G. and Hood, C. (2006) 'Have targets improved performance in the English NHS?', *British Medical Journal*, 332, pp 419-22.

Bird, S. M., Cox, D., Farewell, V. T., Goldstein, H., Holt, T. and Smith, P. C. (2005) 'Performance indicators: good, bad, and ugly', *Journal of the Royal Statistical Society A*, 168, pp 1-27.

Bjorvatn, K. and Cappelen, A. W. (2004) *Globalisation, Inequality and Redistribution*, CeGE Discussion Paper 33, Göttingen: Georg-August-Universität Göttingen.

Black, D., Morris, J., Smith, C. and Townsend, P. (1980) *Inequalities in health: report of a Research Working Group*, London: Department of Health and Social Security.

Blackman, T. (1991) *Planning Belfast*, Basingstoke: Avebury.

Blackman, T. (1995) *Urban Policy in Practice*, London: Routledge.

Blackman, T. and Harvey, J. (2001) 'Housing renewal and mental health: a case study', *Journal of Mental Health*, 10, pp 571-83.

Blackman, T., Mitchell, L., Burton, E., Jenks, M., Parsons, M., Raman, S. and Williams, K. (2003) 'The accessibility of public spaces for people with dementia: a new priority for the 'open city'', *Disability & Society*, 18 (3), pp 357-71.

Boardman, J. D., Finch, B. K., Ellison, C. G., Williams, D. R. and Jackson, J. S. (2001) 'Neighborhood disadvantage, stress, and drug use among adults', *Journal of Health and Social Behavior*, 42, pp 151-65.

Bonnefoy, X. R., Braubach, M., Moissonnier, B., Monolbaev, K. and Röbbel, N. (2003) 'Housing and health in Europe: preliminary results of a Pan-European Study', *American Journal of Public Health*, 93, pp 1559-63.

Bourdieu, P. (1977) *Outline of a Theory of Practice*, Cambridge: Cambridge University Press.

British Medical Journal (2003) *Housing and Health: Building for the Future*, London: British Medical Association.

Brune, N. and Garrett, G. (2005) 'The globalization Rorschach Test: international economic integration, inequality, and the role of government', *Annual Review of Political Science*, 8, pp 399-423.

Brunner, E. (1996) 'The social and biological basis of cardiovascular disease in office workers', in D. Blane, E. Brunner and R. Wilkinson (eds), *Health and Social Organization*, London: Routledge, pp 272-302.

Buchanan, M. (2002) *Nexus: Small Worlds and the Groundbreaking Science of Networks*, London: W. W. Norton & Co.

Bundred, S. (2005) 'Minimizing the burden of regulation', *Review: The Newsletter of the Public Management and Policy Association*, 28, p 14.

Burningham, K. and Thrush, D. (2003) 'Experiencing environmental inequality: the everyday concerns of disadvantaged groups', *Housing Studies*, 18 (4), pp 517-36.

Burns, W. (1963) *New Towns for Old: The Technique of Urban Renewal*, London: Leonard Hill Ltd.

Buron, L. (2004) *An Improved Living Environment? Neighborhood Outcomes for HOPE VI Relocatees*, Washington, DC: The Urban Institute.

Burrows, R., Ellison, N. and Woods, B. (2005) *Sorted? Internet-based Neighbourhood Information Systems and their Consequences*, York: Joseph Rowntree Foundation.

Byrne, D. (1998) *Complexity Theory and the Social Sciences*, London: Routledge.

Byrne, D. (1999) *Social Exclusion*, Buckingham: Open University Press.

Byrne, D. (2002) *Interpreting Quantitative Data*, London: Sage Publications.

Cabinet Office (1999) *Modernising Government*, Cmnd 4310, London: The Stationery Office.

Cabinet Office (2005) *Improving the Prospects of People Living in Areas of Multiple Deprivation in England*, London: Prime Minister's Strategy Unit.

Callaghan, P. and Morrissey, J. (1993) 'Social support and health: a review', *Journal of Advanced Nursing*, 18, pp 203-10.

Chandola, T., Clarke, P. and Bartley, M. (2005) 'Who you live with and where you live: setting the context for health using multiple membership multilevel models', *Journal of Epidemiology and Community Health*, 59, pp 170-5.

Chapman, J. (2004) *System Failure: Why Governments Must Learn to Think Differently* (2nd edition), London: Demos.

Chisholm, J. S. and Burbank, V. K. (2001) 'Evolution and inequality', *International Journal of Epidemiology*, 30, pp 206-11.

Chiu, L. F. (2003) *Inequalities of Access to Cancer Screening: A Literature Review*, Cancer Screening Series No. 1, Sheffield: NHS Cancer Screening Programmes.

Cho, Y., Park, G.-S. and Echevarria-Cruz, S. (2005) 'Perceived neighbourhood characteristics and the health of adult Koreans', *Social Science & Medicine*, 60, pp 1285-97.

Cilliers, P. (1998) *Complexity and Postmodernism*, London: Routledge.

Clarke, M. and Stewart, J. (1997) *Handling the Wicked Issues: A Challenge for Government*, Birmingham: University of Birmingham.

Cohen, D., Spear, S., Scribner, R., Kissinger, P., Mason, K. and Wildgen, J. (2000) '"Broken windows" and the risk of gonorrhea', *American Journal of Public Health*, 90 (2), pp 230-6.

Cohen, D. A., Funch, B. K., Bower, A. and Sastry, N. (2006) 'Collective efficacy and obesity: the potential influence of social factors on health', *Social Science & Medicine*, 62, pp 769-78.

Cole, M. (2003) 'Public property', in *Reducing Health Inequalities: Local Government and the NHS Working Together*, Local Government Chronicle and Health Services Journal special supplement, March, p 14.

Coley, R. L., Kuo, F. E. and Sullivan, W. C. (1997) 'Where does community grow? The social context created by nature in urban public housing', *Environment and Behavior*, 29 (4), pp 468-94.

Collinge, A., Duffy, B. and Page, B. (2005) *Physical Capital: Liveability in 2005*, London: MORI.

Commission on Social Justice (1994) *Social Justice, Strategies for National Renewal: Report of the Commission on Social Justice*, London: Vintage.

Community Development Project (1977) *Gilding the Ghetto: The State and the Poverty Experiments*, London: CDP.

Coote, A. (ed) (2002) *Claiming the Health Dividend: Unlocking the Benefits of NHS Spending*, London: King's Fund.

Coote, A., Allen, J. and Woodhead, D. (2004) *Finding out What Works*, London: King's Fund.

Craig, N., Wright, B., Hanlon, P. and Galbraith, S. (2006) 'Does health care improve health?', *Journal of Health Services Research & Policy*, 11 (1), pp 1-2.

CRESR (Centre for Regional, Economic and Social Research) (2005) *Research Report 17: New Deal for Communities 2001-2005: An Interim Evaluation*, London: ODPM.

Crisp, N. (2003) *Chief Executive's Report to the NHS*, London: Department of Health.

Crow, G. (2002) 'Community studies: fifty years of theorization', *Sociological Research Online*, 7 (3), www.socresonline.org.uk/7/3/crow.html

Cummins, S. and Macintyre, S. (2002) '"Food deserts" – evidence and assumption in health policy making', *British Medical Journal*, 325, pp 436-8.

Curtis, L. J., Dooley, M. D. and Phipps, S. A. (2004) 'Child well-being and neighbourhood quality: evidence from the Canadian National Longitudinal Survey of Children and Youth', *Social Science & Medicine*, 58, pp 1917-27.

Curtis, S., Southall, H., Congdon, P. and Dodgeon, B. (2004) 'Area effects on health variation over the life-course: analysis of the longitudinal study sample in England using new data on area of residence in childhood', *Social Science & Medicine*, 58, pp 57-74.

Davey-Smith, G., Ebrahim, S. and Frankel, S. (2001) 'How policy informs the evidence', *British Medical Journal*, 322, pp 184-5.

Davis, H., Downe, J. and Martin, S. (2001) *External Inspection of Local Government: Driving Improvement or Drowning in Detail?*, York: Joseph Rowntree Foundation.

Day, K., Carreon, D. and Stump, C. (2000) 'The therapeutic design of environments for people with dementia: a review of the empirical research', *The Gerontologist*, 40 (4), pp 397-416.

De Silva, M. J., McKenzie, K., Harpham, T. and Huttly, S. R. A. (2005) 'Social capital and mental illness: a systematic review', *Journal of Epidemiology and Community Health*, 59, pp 619-27.

de Vries, D., Verheij, R. A., Groenewegen, P. P. and Spreeuwenberg, P. (2003) 'Natural environments – healthy environments? An exploratory analysis of the relationship between greenspace and health', *Environment and Planning A*, 35, pp 1717-31.

Deeming, C. (2005) 'Keeping health on a minimum wage', *British Medical Journal*, 331, pp 857-8.

Dembski, W. A. (2003) 'Can evolutionary algorithms generate specified complexity?', in N. H. Gregersen (ed) *From Complexity to Life*, Oxford: Oxford University Press, pp 93-113.

DETR (Department of the Environment, Transport and the Regions) (2000) *Tomorrow's Roads: Safer for Everyone*, London: DETR.

DfES (Department for Education and Skills) (2004) *Statistics for Education: Variation in Pupil Progress 2003*, Issue No. 02/04, London: HMSO.

DfES (2005) *Youth Matters*, Cm 6629, London: HMSO.

DfT (Department for Transport) (2002) *Child Road Safety: Achieving the 2010 Target*, London: DfT.

DfT (2004) *Tomorrow's Roads – Safer for Everyone: The First Three Year Review*, London: DfT.

DH (Department of Health) (1992) *The Health of the Nation*, London: HMSO.

DH (1998) *Our Healthier Nation*, London: The Stationery Office.

DH (2000a) *Health Survey for England 1999: The Health of Minority Ethnic Groups*, London: The Stationery Office.

DH (2000b) *The NHS Plan*, London: HMSO.

DH (2003) *Tackling Health Inequalities: A Programme for Action*, London: DH.

DH (2004a) *Choosing Health*, Cm 6374, London: The Stationery Office.

DH (2004b) *National Standards, Local Action: Health and Social Care Standards and Planning Framework*, London: DH.

DH (2005a) *Tackling Health Inequalities: Status Report on the Programme for Action*, London: DH.

DH (2005b) *Tackling Health Inequalities: The Spearhead Group of Local Authorities and Primary Care Trusts*, London: DH.

DH (2005c) *Tackling Health Inequalities: What Works*, Best Practice Guidance, London: DH.

DH (2005d) *Delivering Choosing Health: Making Healthier Choices Easier*, London: DH.

DH (2006a) *The NHS in England: The Operating Framework for 2006/7*, London: DH.

DH (2006b) *Our Health, Our Care, Our Say: A New Direction for Community Services*, Cm 6737, London: The Stationery Office.

Dorling, D. and Rees, P. (2003) 'A nation still dividing: the British census and social polarisation 1971-2001', *Environment and Planning A*, 35, pp 1287-1313.

Drucker, P. (1954) *The Principles of Management*, New York: Harper & Row.

Drukker, M., Feron, F. J. M. and van Os, J. (2004) 'Income inequality at neighbourhood level and quality of life – a contextual analysis', *Social Psychiatry and Psychiatric Epidemiology*, 39 (6), pp 457-63.

Drukker, M., Kaplan, C., Feron, F. and van Os, J. (2003) 'Children's health-related quality of life, neighbourhood socio-economic deprivation and social capital: a contextual analysis', *Social Science and Medicine*, 57, pp 825-41.

Duncan, C., Jones, K. and Moon, G. (1999) 'Smoking and deprivation: are there neighbourhood effects?', *Social Science & Medicine*, 48, pp 497-505.

Ecotec Research & Consulting Ltd (2005) *Understanding the Drivers of Housing Market Change in the New Heartlands Housing Market Renewal Area*, Birmingham: Ecotec.

Ellaway, A. and Macintyre, S. (2001) 'Women in their place: gender and perceptions of neighborhoods in the West of Scotland', in I. Dyck, N. Davis Lewis and S. McLafferty (eds) *Geographies of Women's Health*, London: Routledge, pp 265-81.

Ellaway, A., Macintyre, S. and Bonnefoy, X. (2005) 'Graffiti, greenery, and obesity in adults: secondary analysis of European cross sectional survey', *British Medical Journal*, 331, pp 611-12.

Elliott, M. (2000) 'The stress process in neighbourhood context', *Health & Place*, 6, pp 287-9.

Ellison, N. (2005) *The Transformation of Welfare States?*, London: Routledge.

Evans, J., Hyndman, S., Stewart-Brown, S., Smith, D. and Petersen, S. (2000) 'An epidemiological study of the relative importance of damp housing in relation to adult health', *Journal of Epidemiology and Community Health*, 54, pp 677-86.

Eve, R. A., Horsfall, S. and Lee, M. E. (eds) (1997) *Chaos, Complexity, and Sociology*, London: Sage Publications.

Farrington-Douglas, J. and Allen, J. (2005) *Equitable Choices for Health*, London: IPPR.

Field, K. S. and Briggs, D. J. (2001) 'Socio-economic and locational determinants of accessibility and utilization', *Health and Social Care in the Community*, 9 (5), pp 294-308.

Fitz-Gibbon, C. T. (1996) *Monitoring Education*, London: Cassell.

Fleetcroft, R. and Cookson, R. (2006) 'Do the incentive payments in the new NHS contract for primary care reflect likely population health gains?', *Journal of Health Services Research and Policy*, 11 (1), pp 27-31.

Fontaine, H. and Gourlet, Y. (1997) 'Fatal pedestrian accidents in France: a typological analysis', *Accident Analysis and Prevention*, 29, pp 303-12.

Foster, C., Hillsdon, M. and Thorogood, M. (2004) 'Environmental perceptions and walking in English adults', *Journal of Epidemiology and Community Health*, 58, pp 924-8.

Freeman, K. (2004) 'Veg and the City', *Housing Today*, 12 March.

Freisthler, B., Lascala, E. A., Gruenewald, P. J. and Treno, A. J. (2005) 'An examination of drug activity: effects of neighborhood social organization on the development of drug distribution systems', *Substance Use & Misuse*, 40 (5), pp 671-86.

Galea, S., Rudenstine, S. and Vlahov, D. (2005) 'Drug use, misuse, and the urban environment', *Drug and Alcohol Review*, 24, pp 127-36.

Ganz, M. L. (2000) 'The relationship between external threats and smoking in Central Harlem', *American Journal of Public Health*, 90, pp 367-71.

Gatrell, A. C. (2005) 'Complexity theory and geographies of health: a critical assessment', *Social Science & Medicine*, 60, pp 2661-71.

Gatrell, A. C., Popay, J. and Thomas, C. (2004) 'Mapping the determinants of health inequalities in social space: can Bourdieu help us?', *Health & Place*, 10, pp 245-57.

GFA Consulting (2005) *Improving Floor Target Performance: What works?*, London: ODPM.

Gilbert, N. and Troitzsch, K. G. (1999) *Simulation for the Social Scientist*, Buckingham: Open University Press.

Giles-Corti, B. and Donovan, R. J. (2002) 'Socioeconomic status differences in recreational physical activity levels and real and perceived access to a supportive physical environment', *Preventive Medicine*, 35 (6), pp 601-11.

Giles-Corti, B., Broomhall, M. H., Knuiman, M., Collins, C., Douglas, K., Lange, A. and Donovan, R. J. (2005) 'Increasing walking: how important is distance to, attractiveness, and size of public open space?', *American Journal of Preventative Medicine*, 28, pp 169-76.

Gilleard, C. and Higgs, P. (2005) *Contexts of Ageing*, Cambridge: Polity.

Gladwell, M. (2000) *The Tipping Point: How Little Things can make a Big Difference*, London: Abacus.

Glass, T. A. and Balfour, J. L. (2003) 'Neighborhoods, aging, and functional limitation', in I. Kawachi and L. Berkman (eds) *Neighborhoods and Health*, Oxford: Oxford University Press, pp 303-34.

Goldsmith, A. H., Veum, J. R. and Darity, W. (1995) 'Are being unemployed and being out of the labor-force distinct states – a psychological approach', *Journal of Economic Psychology*, 16, pp 275-95.

Graham, H. and McDermott, E. (2006) 'Qualitative research and the evidence base of policy: insights from studies of teenage mothers in the UK', *Journal of Social Policy*, 35 (1), pp 21-37.

Green, G., Grimsley, M. and Stafford, B. (2005) *The Dynamics Of Neighbourhood Sustainability*, York: Joseph Rowntree Foundation.

Greer, S. (2006) 'The politics of health-policy divergence', in J. Adams and K. Schmueker (eds) *Devolution in Practice 2006: Public Policy Differences within the UK*, Newcastle Upon Tyne: IPPR North.

Gregersen, N. H. (ed) (2003) *From Complexity to Life: On the Emergence of Life and Meaning*, Oxford: Oxford University Press.

Halliday, J. and Asthana, S. (2005) 'Policy at the margins: developing community capacity in a rural Health Action Zone', *Area*, 37 (2), pp 180-8.

Hamer, L. (2004) *Improving Patient Access to Health Services: A National Review and Case Studies of Current Approaches*, London: Health Development Agency.

Hamilton, C. (2003) *Growth Fetish*, London: Pluto Press.

Harris, T. (2001) 'Recent developments in understanding the psychosocial aspects of depression', *British Medical Bulletin*, 57, pp 17-32.

Harrison, C. S., Grant, M. and Conway, B. A. (2004) 'Haptic interfaces for wheelchair navigation in the built environment', *Presence*, 13 (5), pp 520-34.

Harrison, S. and Wood, B. (1999) 'Designing health service organization in the UK, 1968 to 1998: from blueprint to bright idea and "manipulated emergence"', *Public Administration*, 77, pp 751-68.

Hastings, A., Flint, J., McKenzie, C. and Mills, C. (2005) *Cleaning up Neighbourhoods: Environmental Problems and Service Provision in Deprived Areas*, Bristol: The Policy Press.

Health Committee (2004) *Obesity: Third Report of Session 2003-04*, Vol 1, HC 23-1, London: The Stationery Office.

Healthcare Commission (2005a) *State of Healthcare 2005*, London: Healthcare Commission.

Healthcare Commission (2005b) *Assessment for Improvement: The Annual Health Check*, London: Healthcare Commission.

Healthcare Commission, Audit Commission, Commission for Social Care Inspection, Health & Safety Executive, Mental Health Act Commission, National Audit Office, NHS Estates, NHS Litigation Authority and Postgraduate Medical Education and Training Board (2004) *Concordat between Bodies Inspecting, Regulating and Auditing Healthcare*, June, London: Healthcare Commission.

Healthier Neighbourhoods Action Team (2005) *Getting Started on Health: An Action Guide*, London: Neighbourhood Management National Network.

Hembree, C., Galea, S., Ahern, J., Tracy, M., Piper, T. M., Miller, J., Vlahov, D. and Tardiff, K. J. (2005) 'The urban built environment and overdose mortality in New York city neighborhoods', *Health & Place*, 11 (2), pp 147-56.

Heslop, P., Smith, G. D., Carroll, D., Macleod, J., Hyland, F. and Hart, C. (2001) 'Perceived stress and coronary heart disease risk factors: the contribution of socio-economic position', *British Journal of Health Psychology*, 6 (2), pp 167-78.

Hill, T. D. and Angel, R. J. (2005) 'Neighborhood disorder, psychological distress, and heavy drinking', *Social Science & Medicine*, 61, pp 965-75.

HM Treasury (2004) *Spending Review: New Public Spending Plans 2005-2008*, Cm 6237, London: The Stationery Office.

HM Treasury (2005) *Pre-Budget Report*, Cm 6701, London: HMSO.

Holmes, C. (2006) *Mixed Communities: Success and Sustainability*, York: Joseph Rowntree Foundation.

Hood, C. (2001) 'Public service managerialism: onwards and upwards, or 'Trobriand cricket' again?', *The Political Quarterly*, 72 (3), pp 300-9.

Hudson, B. and Henwood, M. (2002) 'The NHS and social care: the final countdown?', *Policy & Politics*, 30 (2), pp 153-66.

Ittelson, W. H. (1973) *Environment and Cognition*, New York: Seminar Press.

Jackson, B. and Segal, P. (2004) *Why Inequality Matters*, London: Catalyst.

Jackson, L. E. (2003) 'The relationship of urban design to human health and condition', *Landscape and Urban Planning*, 64, pp 191-200.

Jacobson, J. O. (2004) 'Place and attrition from substance abuse treatment', *Journal of Drug Issues*, 34 (1), pp 23-49.

Jain, A. (2006) 'Treating obesity in individuals and populations', *British Medical Journal*, 331, pp 1387-90.

Judge, K. and Bauld, L. (2005) 'Conclusion', in M. Barnes, L. Bauld, M. Benzeval, K. Judge, M. Mackenzie and H. Sullivan (2005) *Health Action Zones: Partnerships for Health Equity*, London: Routledge, pp 185-99.

Judge, K., Barnes, M., Bauld, L., Benzeval, M., Killoran, A., Robinson, R., Wigglesworth, R. and Zeilig, H. (1999) *Health Action Zones: Learning to Make a Difference*, Canterbury: Personal Social Services Research Unit, University of Kent.

Kadushin, C., Reber, E., Saxe, L. and Livert, D. (1998) 'The substance use system: social and neighbourhood environments associated with substance use and misuse', *Substance Use & Misuse*, 33 (8), pp 1681-710.

Kaplan, R. and Kaplan, S. (1989) *The Experience of Nature: A Psychological Perspective*, New York: Cambridge University Press.

Kavanagh, D. and Richards, D. (2001) 'Departmentalism and joined-up government: back to the future?', *Parliamentary Affairs*, 54 (1), pp 1-18.

Kawachi, I. and Berkman, L. F. (eds) (2003) *Neighborhoods and Health*, Oxford: Oxford University Press.

Kelso, J. A. S. (1999) *Dynamic Patterns: The Self-Organization of Brain and Behavior*, Cambridge, MA: The MIT Press.

King, W. C., Brach, J. S., Belle, S., Killingworth, R., Fenton, M. and Kriska, A. M. (2003) 'The relationship between convenience of destination and walking levels in older women', *American Journal of Health Promotion*, 18 (1), pp 74-82.

Kintrea, K. and Morgan, J. (2005) *Evaluation of English Housing Policy 1975-2000*, London: ODPM.

Kitwood, T. (1997) *Dementia Reconsidered*, Buckingham: Open University Press.

Kleinschmidt, I., Hills, M. and Elliott, P. (1995) 'Smoking behaviour can be predicted by neighbourhood deprivation measures', *Journal of Epidemiology & Community Health*, 49, S72-S77.

Kling, J. R., Liebman, J. B. and Katz, L. F. (2005) 'Experimental analysis of neighborhood effects', available at: http://nber.org/~kling/mto/mto_exp.pdf (accessed 25 September 2005).

Kobetz, E., Daniel, M. and Earp, J. A. (2003) 'Neighborhood poverty and self-reported health among low-income, rural women, 50 years and older', *Health & Place*, 9 (3), pp 263-71.

Kooiman, J. (2003) *Governing as Governance*, London: Sage Publications.

Kreuter, M. W., De Rosa, C., Howze, E. H. and Baldwin, G. T. (2004) 'Understanding wicked problems: a key to advancing environmental health promotion', *Health Education & Behavior*, 31 (4), pp 441-54.

Kunst, A. E., Bos, V., Lahelma, E., Bartley, M., Lissau, I., Regidor, E., Mielck, A., Cardano, M., Dalstra, J. A. A., Geurts, J. J. M., Helmert, U., Lennartsson, C., Ramm, J., Spadea, T., Stronegger, W. J. and Mackenbach, J. P. (2005) 'Trends in socioeconomic inequalities in self-assessed health in 10 European countries', *International Journal of Epidemiology*, 34, pp 295-305.

Kuo, F. E. and Sullivan, W. C. (2001a) 'Environment and crime in the inner city – does vegetation reduce crime?', *Environment and Behavior*, 33 (3), pp 343-67.

Kuo, F. E. and Sullivan, W. C. (2001b) 'Aggression and violence in the inner city – effects of environment via mental fatigue', *Environment and Behavior*, 33 (4), pp 543-71.

Kuo, F. E., Sullivan, W. C., Coley, R. L. and Brunson, L. (1998) 'Fertile ground for community: inner-city neighborhood common spaces', *American Journal of Community Psychology*, 26 (6), pp 823-51.

Lader, D. and Meltzer, H. (2003) *Smoking Related Behaviour and Attitudes 2002*, London: Office for National Statistics.

Larson, E. B., Wang, L., Bowen, J. D., McCormick, W. C., Teri, L., Crane, P. and Kukull, W. (2006) 'Exercise is associated with reduced risk for incident dementia among persons 65 years of age and older', *Annals of Internal Medicine*, 144, pp 73-81.

Lash, S. and Urry, J. (1987) *The End of Organized Capitalism*, Cambridge: Polity.

Latkin, C. A. and Curry, A. D. (2003) 'Stressful neighborhoods and depression: a prospective study of the impact of neighborhood disorder', *Journal of Health & Social Behavior*, 44, pp 34-44.

Law, M., Wilson, K., Eyles, J., Elliott, S., Jerrett, M., Moffatt, T. and Luginaah, I. (2005) 'Meeting health need, assessing health care: the role of neighbourhood', *Health & Place*, 11, pp 367-77.

Lawlor, D. A., Frankel, S., Shaw, M., Ebrahim, S. and Smith, G.D. (2003) 'Smoking and ill health: does lay epidemiology explain the failure of smoking cessation programs among deprived population?', *American Journal of Public Health*, 93, pp 266-70.

Lawton, M. P. (1980) *Environment and Aging*, Belmont, CA: Brooks-Cole.

Lawton, M. P. (1982) 'Competence, environmental press, and the adaptation of older people', in M. P. Lawton, P. Windley and T. Byertss (eds) *Aging and the Environment: Theoretical Approaches*, New York: Springer, pp 33-59.

Lawton, M. P. (1989) 'Three functions of the residential environment', *Journal of Housing for the Elderly*, 5, pp 35-50.

Lawton, M. P. (1998) 'Environment and aging: theory revisited', in R. Scheidt and P. Windley (eds) *Environment and Aging Theory*, Westport, CT: Greenwood Press, pp 1-32.

Layard, R. (2005) *Happiness: Lessons from a New Science*, London: Allen Lane.

Leclerc, A., Chastang, J.-F., Menvielle, G. and Luce, D. (2006) 'Socioeconomic inequalities in premature mortality in France: have they widened in recent decades?', *Social Science & Medicine*, 62, pp 2035-45.

Lee, P. and Nevin, B. (2003) 'Changing demand for housing: restructuring markets and the public policy framework', *Housing Studies*, 18 (1), pp 65-86.

Lefebvre, H. (2000) *La Production de l'Espace* (4th edition), Paris: Anthropos.

Levin, K. A. and Leyland, A. H. (2006) 'A comparison of health inequalities in urban and rural Scotland', *Social Science & Medicine*, 62, pp 1457-64.

Leyland, A. H. (2005) 'Socioeconomic gradients in the prevalence of cardiovascular disease in Scotland: the roles of composition and context', *Journal of Epidemiology and Community Health*, 59, pp 799-803.

Lindström, M. (2003) 'Social capital and sense of insecurity in the neighbourhood: a population-based multilevel analysis in Malmo, Sweden', *Social Sciences & Medicine*, 56, pp 1111-20.

Lindström, M. and The Malmö Shoulder-Neck Study Group (2006) 'Psychosocial work conditions, social participation and social capital: a causal pathway investigated in a longitudinal study', *Social Science & Medicine*, 62 (2), pp 280-91.

Lipsitz, L. A. and Goldberger, A. L. (1992) 'Loss of 'complexity' and aging', *Journal of the American Medical Association*, 267 (13), pp 1806-9.

Liverpool City Council (with partners) (2004) *Health Impact Assessment of Liverpool City Council's Housing Strategy Statement: Final Report 2003*, Liverpool: Liverpool City Council.

Long, D. (2001) *A Toolkit of Sustainability Indicators*, London: The Housing Corporation and the European Institute for Urban Affairs, Liverpool John Moores University.

Lorimer, K. (2004) 'Residents are more dissatisfied', *Local Government Chronicle*, 2, p 2.

Low, A. and Low, A. (2006) 'Importance of relative measures in policy on health inequalities', *British Medical Journal*, 332, pp 967-9.

Luhmann, N. (1995) *Social Systems*, Stanford, CA: Stanford University Press.

Lupton, R. (2003) *'Neighbourhood Effects': Can we Measure them and does it Matter?*, London: Centre for the Analysis of Social Exclusion, London School of Economics and Political Science.

Lyons, M. (Chair) (2006) *National Prosperity, Local Choice and Civic Engagement*, London: HMSO.

MacDonald, R. and Marsh, J. (2005) *Disconnected Youth? Growing Up in Britain's Poor Neighbourhoods*, London: Palgrave.

Macintyre, K., Stewart, S., Chalmers, J., Pell, J., Finlayson, A., Boyd, J., Redpath, A., McMurray, J. and Capewell, S. (2001) 'Relation between socioeconomic deprivation and death from a first myocardial infarction in Scotland: population based analysis', *British Medical Journal*, 322, pp 1152-3.

Macintyre, S. and Ellaway, A. (2003) 'Neighborhoods and health: an overview', in I. Kawachi and L. F. Berkman (eds) *Neighborhoods and Health*, Oxford: Oxford University Press, pp 20-42.

Macintyre, S., Maciver, S. and Sooman, A. (1993) 'Area, class and health: should we be focusing on places or people?', *Journal of Social Policy*, 22, pp 213-33.

Macintyre, S., Hiscock, R., Kearns, A. and Ellaway, A. (2001) 'Housing tenure and car access: further exploration of the nature of their relations with health in a UK setting', *Journal of Epidemiology and Community Health*, 55, pp 330-1.

Mackenbach, J. and Bakker, M. (eds) (2002) *Reducing Inequalities in Health: A European Perspective*, London: Routledge.

Macleod, J., Smith, G. D., Metcalfe, C. and Hart, C. (2005) 'Is subjective social status a more important determinant of health than objective social status? Evidence from a prospective observational study of Scottish men', *Social Science & Medicine*, 61, pp 1916-29.

Marchand, A., Demers, A. and Durand, P. (2005) 'Does work really cause distress? The contribution of occupational structure and work organization to the experience of psychological distress', *Social Science & Medicine*, 61, pp 1-14.

Marmot, M. (2004) *Status Syndrome*, London: Bloomsbury.

Marsh, A., Gordon, D., Pantazis, C. and Heslop, P. (1999) *Home Sweet Home? The Impact of Poor Housing on Health*, Bristol: The Policy Press.

McCulloch, A. (2006) 'Variation in children's cognitive and behavioural adjustment between different types of place in the British National Child Development Study', *Social Science & Medicine*, 62, pp 1865-79.

McKeown, T. (1979) *The Role of Medicine*, Oxford: Blackwell.

McKie, L., Laurier, E., Taylor, R. J. and Lennox, A. S. (2003) 'Eliciting the smoker's agenda: implications for policy and practice', *Social Science & Medicine*, 56, pp 83-94.

Mclean, C., Carmona, C., Francis, S., Wohlgemuth, C. and Mulvihill, C. (2005) *Worklessness and Health – What do we Know about the Causal Relationship?*, London: Health Development Agency.

McLoone, P. (2001) 'Targeting deprived areas within small areas in Scotland: population study', *British Medical Journal*, 323, pp 374-5.

McLoone, P. and Ellaway, A. (1999) 'Postcodes don't indicate individuals' social class', *British Medical Journal*, 319, p 1003.

Meen, G., Gibb, K., Goody, J., McGarth, T. and Mackinnon, J. (2005) *Economic Segregation in England: Causes, Consequences and Policy*, Bristol: The Policy Press.

Millward, L. (2005) "We are announcing your target': reflections on performance language in the making of English housing policy', *Local Government Studies*, 31, pp 597-614.

Milne, E. (2005) 'NHS smoking cessation services and smoking prevalence: observational study', *British Medical Journal*, 330, p 760.

Mitchell, L., Burton, E., Raman, S., Blackman, T., Jenks, M. and Williams, K. (2003) 'Making the outside world dementia-friendly: design issues and considerations', *Environment and Planning B: Planning and Design*, 30, pp 605-32.

Mitchell, R. D., Dorling, D. and Shaw, M. (2000) *Inequalities in Life and Death*, Bristol: The Policy Press.

Mohan, J., Twigg, L., Barnard, S. and Jones, K. (2005) 'Social capital, geography and health: a small-area analysis for England', *Social Science & Medicine*, 60, pp 1267-83.

Monden, C. W. S., van Lenthe, F. J. and Mackenbach, J. P. (forthcoming) 'A simultaneous analysis of neighbourhood and childhood socio-economic environment with self-assessed health and health-related behaviours', *Health & Place*.

Moobela, C. (2005) 'From worst slum to best example of regeneration: complexity in the regeneration of Hulme, Manchester', *Emergence: Complexity and Organization*, 7 (1), pp 29-42.

Mooney, G. and Scott, G. (eds) (2005) *Exploring Social Policy in the 'New' Scotland*, Bristol: The Policy Press.

Moran, M. (2001) 'The rise of the regulatory state in Britain', *Parliamentary Affairs*, 54 (1), pp 19-34.

MORI (2002) *The Rising Prominence of Liveability or are we Condemned to a Life of Grime?*, London: MORI publications.

Morris, J. N., Donkin, A. J. M., Wonderling, D., Wilkinson, P. and Dowler, E. (2000) 'A minimum income for healthy living', *Journal of Epidemiology and Community Health*, 54, pp 885-9.

Mulgan, G. and Bury, F. (2006) *Double Devolution: the renewal of local government*, London: The Smith Institute.

Naderi, J. R. and Raman, B. (2005) 'Capturing impressions of pedestrian landscapes used for healing purposes with decision tree learning', *Landscape and Urban Planning*, 73, pp 155-66.

NAO (National Audit Office) (2001) *Tackling Obesity in England*, London: NAO.

NAO (2005) *Innovation in the NHS: Local Improvement Finance Trusts*, London: NAO.

National Housing Law Project, Poverty & Race Research Action Council, Sherwood Research Associates and ENPHRONT (2002) *False HOPE: A Critical Assessment of the HOPE VI Public Housing Redevelopment Program*, Oakland, CA: National Housing Law Project.

Nevin, B., Lee, P., Goodson, L., Murie, A. and Phillimore, J. (2001) *Changing Housing Markets and Urban Regeneration in the M62 Corridor*, Birmingham: Centre for Urban and Regional Studies, University of Birmingham.

Newman, J. (2001) *Modernising Governance*, London: Sage Publications.

NHS Health and Social Care Information Centre (2005) *Health Survey for England 2004 – Updating of Trend Tables to Include 2004 Data*, London: Health and Social Care Information Centre.

NHS Modernisation Board (2004) *Caring in Many Ways: Annual Report 2004*, London: The Stationery Office.

Niggebrugge, A., Haynes, R., Jones, A., Lovett, A. and Harvey, I. (2005) 'The index of multiple deprivation 2000 access domain: a useful indicator for public health?', *Social Science & Medicine*, 60, pp 2743-53.

Nolte, E. and McKee, M. (2004) *Does Health Care Save Lives?*, London: The Nuffield Trust.

Norman, P., Boyle, P. and Rees, P. (2005) 'Selective migration, health and deprivation: a longitudinal analysis', *Social Science & Medicine*, 60, pp 2755-71.

NEHB (North East Housing Board) (2005) *A New Housing Strategy for the North East*, Newcastle Upon Tyne: NEHB.

NRU (Neighbourhood Renewal Unit) (2004) *The Places Project Interim Report*, London: ODPM.

NRU (2005a) *Smarter Delivery, Better Neighbourhoods*, London: ODPM.

NRU (2005b) *Creating Healthier Communities: A Resource Pack for Local Partnerships*, London: ODPM and Department of Health.

NRU Health Team (2006) Policy Update, January.

Oakes, J. M. (2004) 'The (mis)estimation of neighborhood effects: causal inference for a practicable social epidemiology', *Social Science & Medicine*, 58, pp 1929-52.

ODPM (Office of the Deputy Prime Minister) (2003a) *Sustainable Communities: Building for the Future*, London: ODPM.

ODPM (2003b) *English House Condition Survey 2001*, London: HMSO.

ODPM (2004) *A Decent Home: The Definition and Guidance for Implementation*, London: ODPM.

ODPM (2005a) 'Government allocates £1.3 billion to local authorities in greatest need to improve quality of life', News Release, 21 July.

ODPM (2005b) *Making it Happen in Deprived Neighbourhoods*, London: ODPM.

ODPM (2005c) *Sustainable Communities: People, Places and Prosperity*, Cm 6425, London: The Stationery Office.

ODPM (2005d) *Citizen Engagement and Public Services: Why Neighbourhoods Matter*, London: ODPM.

ODPM (2005e) *Local Strategic Partnerships: Shaping their Future*, London: ODPM.

ODPM/Home Office (2005) *Citizen Engagement and Public Services: Why Neighbourhoods Matter*, London: The Stationery Office.

ODPM/Housing, Planning, Local Government and the Regions Committee (2004) *Fifth Report: Session 2003-04*, London: HMSO.

OECD (Organisation for Economic Co-operation and Development) (2005) *Society at a Glance: OECD Social Indicators*, Paris: OECD Publishing.

Office of Public Management, University of the West of England and University of Warwick (2005) *A Process Evaluation of the Negotiation of Pilot Local Area Agreements*, London: ODPM.

Öhlander, E., Vikstrom, M., Lindstrom, M. and Sundquist, K. (2006) 'Neighbourhood non-employment and daily smoking: a population-based study of women and men in Sweden', *European Journal of Public Health*, 16, pp 78-84.

One City Partnership Nottingham (2004) *OCPN Improvement Plan 2004/2005 – Draft Floor Target Action Plan for Health*, Nottingham: OCPN.

ONS (Office for National Statistics) (2005a) *Life Expectancy at Birth by Health and Local Authorities in the United Kingdom 1991-1993 to 2002-2004*, London: ONS.

ONS (2005b) 'Alcohol-related deaths: rates continue to rise', www.statistics.gov.uk/CCI/nugget.asp?ID=1091&Pos=3&ColRank=1&Rank=192 (accessed 6 May 2006).

Ormerod, P. (1997) 'Stopping crime spreading', *New Economy*, 4 (2), pp 83-8.

Orpwood, R., Bjørneby, S., Hagen, I., Mäki, O., Faulkner, R. and Topo, P. (2004) 'User involvement in dementia product development', *Dementia*, 3 (3), pp 263-79.

Page, B. (2003) 'MORI Social Research Institute looks at satisfaction with standard of living and the local area', *Local Government Chronicle*, 7056, p 26.

Palmer, G., Carr, G. and Kenway, P. (2005) *Monitoring Poverty and Social Exclusion 2005*, York: Joseph Rowntree Foundation.

Pantazis, C. (2000) 'Tackling inequalities in crime and social harm', in C. Pantazis and D. Gordon (eds) *Tackling Inequalities: Where Are We Now and What Can Be Done*, Bristol: The Policy Press, pp 117-40.

Pantazis, C. and Gordon, D. (eds) (2000) *Tackling Inequalities: Where Are We Now and What Can Be Done?*, Bristol: The Policy Press.

Parkes, A. and Kearns, A. (2006) 'The multi-dimensional neighbourhood and health: a cross-sectional analysis of the Scottish Household Survey, 2001', *Health & Place*, 12 (1), pp 1-18.

Parks, S. E., Housemann, R.A. and Brownson, R. C. (2003) 'Differential correlates of physical activity in urban and rural adults of various socioeconomic backgrounds in the United States', *Journal of Epidemiology and Community Health*, 57, pp 29-35.

Parsons, T. (1971) *The System of Modern Societies*, Englewood Cliffs, NJ: Prentice-Hall.

Pasaogullari, N. and Doratli, N. (2004) 'Measuring accessibility and utilization of public spaces in Famagusta', *Cities*, 21 (3), pp 225-32.

Paskell, C. and Power, A. (2005) *'The Future's Changed': Local Impacts of Housing, Environment and Regeneration Policy since 1997*, London: Centre for Analysis of Social Exclusion, London School of Economics and Political Science.

Pawson, R. (2002) 'Evidence-based policy: the promise of realist synthesis', *Evaluation*, 8 (3), pp 340-58.

Pawson, R. and Tilley, N. (1997) *Realistic Evaluation*, London: Sage Publications.

Pearl, M. and Pickett, K. E. (2001) 'Explanations for differences in health outcomes between neighbourhoods of varying socioeconomic level: authors' reply', Letters to the Editor, *Journal of Epidemiology and Community Health*, 55, p 847.

Peckham, S. and Exworthy, M. (2003) *Primary Care in the UK: Policy, Organisation and Management*, Basingstoke: Palgrave Macmillan.

Peckham, S., Exworthy, M., Greener, I. and Powell, M. (2005) 'Decentralizing health services: more local accountability or just more central control?', *Public Money & Management*, 25 (4), pp 221-8.

Pickett, K. E., Wakschlag, L. S., Rathouz, P. J., Leventhal, B. L. and Abrams, B. (2002) 'The working-class context of pregnancy smoking', *Health & Place*, 8, pp 167-75.

Plsek, P. (2001) 'Redesigning health care with insights from the science of complex adaptive systems', in Committee on Quality Health Care in America, Institute of Medicine, *Crossing the Quality Chasm: A New Health System for the 21st Century*, Washington, DC: National Academy Press, pp 309-22.

Plsek, P. and Greenhalgh T. (2001) 'The challenge of complexity in health care', *British Medical Journal*, 323, pp 625-8.

Poortinga, W. (2006) 'Social capital: an individual or collective resource for health?', *Social Science & Medicine*, 62 (2), pp 292-302.

Popay, J., Thomas, C., Williams, G., Bennett, S., Gatrell, A. and Bostock, L. (2003) 'A proper place to live: health inequalities, agency and the normative dimensions of space', *Social Science and Medicine*, 57, pp 55-69.

Portugali, J. (ed) (2006) *Complex Artificial Environments*, New York: Springer.

Powell, M.A., Boyne, G. and Ashworth, R. (2001) 'Towards a geography of people poverty and place poverty', *Policy & Politics*, 29 (3), pp 243-58.

Power, C., Bartley, M., Smith, G. D. and Blane, D. (1996) 'Transmission of social and biological risk across the life course', in D. Blane, E. Brunner and R. Wilkinson (eds) *Health and Social Organization: Towards a Health Policy for the 21st Century*, London: Routledge, pp 188-203.

Prime Minister's Strategy Unit (2005) *Improving the Prospects of People Living in Areas of Multiple Deprivation in England*, London: Cabinet Office.

Propper, C., Jones, K., Bolster, A., Burgress, S., Johnston, R. and Sarker, R. (2005) 'Local neighbourhood and mental health: evidence from the UK', *Social Science & Medicine*, 61, pp 2065-83.

Public Administration Select Committee (2003) *On Target? Government by Measurement: The Government's Response to the Committee's Fifth Report*, Sixth Report of Session 2002-03, London: The Stationery Office.

Putnam, R. D. (2000) *Bowling Alone: The Collapse and Revival of American Community*, New York: Simon and Schuster.

Putnam, R. D. and Feldstein, L. M. with Cohen, D. (2003) *Better Together: Restoring the American Community*, London: Simon & Schuster.

Ragin, C. C. (2000) *Fuzzy-set Social Science*, Chicago, IL: University of Chicago Press.

Rashman, L. and Radnor, Z. (2005) 'Learning to improve: approaches to improving local government services', *Public Money & Management*, 25 (1), pp 19-26.

Reeves, D. and Baker, D. (2004) 'Investigating relationships between health need, primary care and social care using routine statistics', *Health & Place*, 10, pp 129-40.

Reijneveld, S. A. (1998) 'The impact of individual and area characteristics on urban socioeconomic differences in health and smoking', *International Journal of Epidemiology*, 27, pp 33-40.

Reijneveld, S.A. (2001) 'Explanations for differences in health outcomes between neighbourhoods of varying socioeconomic level', Letters to the Editor, *Journal of Epidemiology and Community Health*, 55, p 847.

Rittel, H. and Webber, M. (1973) 'Dilemmas in a general theory of planning', *Policy Sciences*, 4, pp 155-69.

Rizzo, A. A., Buckwalter, G. and van der Zaag, C. (2002) 'Virtual environment applications in clinical neuropsychology', in K. M. Stanney (ed) *Handbook of Virtual Environments: Design, Implementation, and Applications*, London: Lawrence Erlbaum Associates, pp 1027-64.

Robinson, F. (1983) 'State planning and spatial change: compromise and contradiction in Peterlee New Town', in J. Anderson, S. Duncan and R. Hudson (eds) *Redundant Spaces in Cities and Regions: Studies in Industrial Decline and Social Change*, London: Academic Press, pp 263-84.

Ropemaker Properties Limited (2005) *Harlow North: The Sustainable Growth of a Town*, Sunbury on Thames: Ropemaker Properties Limited.

Ross, C. E. (2000) 'Walking, exercising, and smoking: does neighborhood matter?', *Social Science & Medicine*, 51, pp 265-74.

Ross, N.A., Dorling, D., Dunn, J. R., Henriksson, G., Glover, J., Lynch, J. and Weitoft, G. R. (2005) 'Metropolitan-income inequality and working-age mortality: a cross-sectional analysis using comparable data from five countries', *Journal of Urban Health: Bulletin of the New York Academy of Medicine*, 82 (1), pp 101-10.

Rudlin, D. and Falk, N. (1999) *Building the 21st Century Home: The Sustainable Urban Neighbourhood*, Oxford: Architectural Press.

Sacker, A., Wiggins, R. D. and Bartley, M. (2006) 'Time and place: putting individual health into context: a multilevel analysis of the British Household Panel Survey, 1991-2001', *Health & Place*, 12 (3), pp 279-90.

Saelens, B. E., Sallis, J. F., Black, J. B. and Chen, D. (2003) 'Neighborhood-based differences in physical activity: an environment scale evaluation', *American Journal of Public Health*, 93, pp 1552-8.

Sælensminde, K. (2004) 'Cost-benefit analyses of walking and cycling track networks taking into account insecurity, health effects and external costs of motorized traffic', *Transportation Research Part A*, 38 (8), pp 593-606.

Scambler, G. (2002) *Health and Social Change*, Buckingham: Open University Press.

Scheidt, R. J. and Windley, P. G. (eds) (2003) *Physical Environments and Aging: Critical Contributions of M. Powell Lawton to Theory and Practice*, New York: The Haworth Press.

Scherder, E. J. A., van Paasschen, J., Deijen, J.-B., van der Knokke, S., Orlebeke, J. F. K., Burgers, I., Devriese, P.-P., Swaab, D. F. and Sergeant, J. A. (2005) 'Physical activity and executive functions in the elderly with mild cognitive impairment', *Aging & Mental Health*, 9 (3), pp 272-80.

Scottish Executive (2005) *Delivering for Health*, Edinburgh: Scottish Executive.

Secretary of State for Health (1998) *Saving Lives: Our Healthier Nation*, London: HMSO.

Secretary of State for Scotland (1999) *Towards a Healthier Scotland*, Cm 4269, Edinburgh: The Stationery Office.

Secretary of State for Wales (1998) *Better Health: Better Wales*, Cm 3922, Cardiff: The Stationery Office.

SEU (Social Exclusion Unit) (1999) *Teenage Pregnancy*, Cm 4342, London: HMSO.

SEU (2001) *A New Commitment to Neighbourhood Renewal: National Strategy Action Plan*, London: Cabinet Office.

SEU (2004) *Mental Health and Social Exclusion*, London: HMSO.

Shannon, C. (2005) 'Race makers', *Local Government Chronicle*, 30 June, pp 24-5.

Shaw, J. (2005) 'Inequality under Labour', *Economic Review*, 23 (2) www.ifs.org.uk/publications.php?publication_id=3530 (accessed 6 May 2006).

Shenassa, E. D., Liebhaber, A. and Ezeamama, A. (2006) 'Perceived safety of area of residence and exercise: a pan-European study', *American Journal of Epidemiology*, 163, pp 1012-17.

Shi, L. and Starfield, B. (2004) 'The effect of primary care physician supply and income inequality on mortality among blacks and whites in US metropolitan areas', *American Journal of Public Health*, 91 (8), pp 1246-50.

Ship, K. M. and Branch, L. G. (1999) 'The Physical Environment as a Determinant of the Health Status of Older Populations', *Canadian Journal on Aging*, 19 (3), pp 313-27.

Shohaimi, S., Luben, R., Wareham, N., Day, N., Bingham, S., Welch, A., Oakes, S. and Khaw, K.-T. (2003) 'Residential area deprivation predicts smoking habit independently of individual educational level and occupational social class: a cross sectional study in the Norfolk cohort of the European Investigation into Cancer (EPIC-Norfolk)', *Journal of Epidemiology and Community Health*, 57, pp 270-6.

Shouls, S., Congdon, P. and Curtis, S. (1996) 'Modelling inequality in reported long term illness in the UK: combining individual and area characteristics', *Journal of Epidemiology and Community Health*, 50, pp 366-76.

Smith, P. C. (2005) 'Performance measurement in health care: history, challenges and prospects', *Public Money and Management*, 25 (3), pp 213-20.

Sooman, A. and Macintyre, S. (1995) 'Health and perceptions of the local environment in socially contrasting neighbourhoods in Glasgow', *Health & Place*, 1, pp 15-26.

SQW Ltd (2006) *Neighbourhood Management – at the Turning Point?*, London: ODPM.

Stacey, R. D. (2003) *Strategic Management and Organisational Dynamics: The Challenge of Complexity*, London: Prentice Hall.

Stafford, M. and Marmot, M. (2003) 'Neighbourhood deprivation and health: does it affect us all equally?', *International Journal of Epidemiology*, 32, pp 357-66.

Stafford, M., Bartley, M., Mitchell, R. and Marmot, M. (2001) 'Characteristics of individuals and characteristics of areas: investigating their influence on health in the Whitehall II study', *Health & Place*, 7, pp 117-29.

Stafford, M., Cummins, S., Macintyre, S., Ellaway, A. and Marmot, N. (2005) 'Gender differences in the associations between health and neighbourhood environment', *Social Science & Medicine*, 60, pp 1681-92.

Stafford, M., Bartley, M., Sacker, A., Marmot, M., Wilkinson, R., Boreham, R. and Thomas, R. (2003) 'Measuring the social environment: social cohesion and material deprivation in English and Scottish neighbourhoods', *Environment and Planning A*, 35, pp 1459-75.

Stead, M., MacAskill, S., MacKintosh, A. M., Reece, J. and Eadie, D. (2001) "It's as if you're locked in': qualitative explanations for area effects on smoking in disadvantaged communities', *Health & Place*, 7, pp 333-43.

Stoker, G. (1998) 'Governance as theory: five propositions', *International Social Science Journal*, 155, pp 17-27.

Sullivan, W. C., Kuo, F. E. and DePooter, S. F. (2004) 'The fruit of urban nature – vital neighborhood spaces', *Environment and Behavior*, 36 (5), pp 678-700.

Sundquist, J., Johansson, S.-E., Yang, M. and Sundquist, K. (2006) 'Low linking social capital as a predictor of coronary heart disease in Sweden: a cohort study of 2.8 million people', *Social Science & Medicine*, 62, pp 954-63.

Sundquist, K., Malmström, M. and Johansson, S.-E. (2004) 'Neighbourhood deprivation and incidence of coronary heart disease: a multilevel study of 2.6 million women and men in Sweden', *Journal of Epidemiology and Community Health*, 58, pp 71-7.

Swann, C., Bowe, K., McCormick, G. and Kosmin, M. (2003) *Teenage Pregnancy and Parenthood: A Review of Reviews*, Evidence Briefing, London: NHS Health Development Agency.

Sweeney, K. and Griffiths, F. (eds) (2002) *Complexity and Healthcare: An introduction*, Abingdon: Radcliffe Medical Press.

Taylor, A. F., Kuo, F. E. and Sullivan, W. C. (2001) 'Coping with ADD – the surprising connection to green play settings', *Environment and Behavior*, 33 (1), pp 54-77.

Taylor, A. F., Kuo, F. E. and Sullivan, W. C. (2002) 'Views of nature and self-discipline: evidence from inner city children', *Journal of Environmental Psychology*, 22 (1-2), pp 49-63.

Taylor, A. F., Wiley, A., Kuo, F. E. and Sullivan, W. C. (1998) 'Growing up in the inner city – green spaces as places to grow', *Environment and Behavior*, 30 (1), pp 3-27.

Taylor, P. J. (1999) 'Places, spaces and Macy's: space–place tensions in the political geographies of modernities', *Progress in Human Geography*, 23 (1), pp 7-26.

Thomas, C., Benzeval, M. and Stansfeld, S. (2005) 'Employment transitions and mental health: an analysis from the British Household Panel Survey', *Journal of Epidemiology and Community Health*, 59, pp 243-9.

Thomas, R., Evans, S., Huxley, P., Gately, C. and Rogers, A. (2005) 'Housing improvement and self-reported mental distress among council estate residents', *Social Science & Medicine*, 60 (12), pp 2773-83.

Thomson, H., Petticrew, M. and Morrison, D. (2002) *Housing Improvement and Health Gain: A Summary and Systematic Review*, Glasgow: MRC Social & Public Health Sciences Unit, University of Glasgow.

Timmins, N. (2005) "Every bit' of NHS spending under review', *Financial Times*, 12 December, p 1.

Tudor Hart, J. (1971) 'The inverse care law', *The Lancet*, 7696, pp 405-12.

Ulrich, R. S. (1984) 'View through a window may influence recovery from surgery', *Science*, 224, pp 420-1.

Unal, B., Alison, J. and Capewell, S. (2005) 'Modelling the decline in coronary heart disease deaths in England and Wales, 1981-2000: comparing contributions from primary prevention and secondary prevention', *British Medical Journal*, 331, p 614.

University of Birmingham School of Public Policy (1999) *Cross-cutting Issues in Public Policy and Public Service*, London: DETR.

Vågerö, D. and Leinsalu, M. (2005) 'Health inequalities and social dynamics in Europe', *British Medical Journal*, 331, pp 186-7.

Vahtera, J., Virtanen, P., Kivimäki, M. and Pentti, J. (1999) 'Workplace as an origin of health inequalities', *Journal of Epidemiology and Community Health*, 53, pp 399-407.

Van Gerven, P. W. M., Pass, F. G. W. C., Van Merrienboer, J. J. G. and Schmidt, H. G. (2000) 'Cognitive load theory and the acquisition of complex cognitive skills in the elderly: towards an integrative framework', *Educational Gerontology*, 26 (6), pp 503-21.

Wahl, H. W. and Weisman, G. D. (2003) 'Environmental gerontology at the beginning of the new millennium: reflections on its historical, empirical, and theoretical development', *Gerontologist*, 43, pp 616-27.

Walrond, S., Natarajan, M. and Chappel, D. (2004) *Premature Mortality from Smoking in the North East of England*, Occasional Paper No. 8, Stockton-on-Tees: North East Public Health Observatory.

Walter, I., Nutley, S. M. and Davies, H. (2005) 'What works to promote evidence-based practice? A cross-sector review', *Evidence & Policy*, 1 (3), pp 335-63.

Wanless, D. (2002) *Securing Our Future Health: Taking a Long-term View*, London: HM Treasury.

Wanless, D. (2004) *Securing Good Health for the Whole Population*, London: HM Treasury.

Weich, S., Burton, E., Blanchard, M., Prince, M., Sproston, K. and Erens, B. (2001) 'Measuring the built environment: validity of a site survey instrument for use in urban settings', *Health & Place*, 7, pp 283-92.

Weiss, L. (2003) 'Introduction: bringing domestic institutions back in', in L. Weiss (ed) *States in the Global Economy*, Cambridge: Cambridge University Press, pp 1-36.

Wells, N. M. (2000) 'At home with nature: effects of 'greenness' on children's cognitive functioning', *Environment and Behavior*, 32 (6), pp 775-95.

Welsh Assembly Government (2005) *Designed for Life: Creating World Class Health and Social Care for Wales in the 21st Century*, Cardiff: Welsh Assembly Government.

Wen, M., Browning, C. R. and Cagney, K. A. (2003) 'Poverty, affluence, and income inequality: neighborhood economic structure and its implications for health', *Social Science & Medicine*, 57, pp 843-60.

Wen, M., Cagney, K. A. and Christakis, N. A. (2005) 'Effect of specific aspects of community social environment on the mortality of individuals diagnosed with serious illness', *Social Science & Medicine*, 61, pp 1119-34.

Weuve, J., Kang, J. H., Manson, J. E., Breteler, M. M. B., Ware, J. H. and Grodstein, F. (2004) 'Physical activity, including walking, and cognitive function in older women', *Journal of the American Medical Association*, 292 (12), pp 1454-61.

Whelan, A., Wrigley, N., Warm, D. and Cannings, E. (2002) 'Life in a "food desert"', *Urban Studies*, 39 (11), pp 2083-2100.

Whitley, R. and Prince, M. (2005) 'Fear of crime, mobility and mental health in inner-city London, UK', *Social Science & Medicine*, 61, pp 1678-88.

Wiggins, M., Rosato, M., Austerberry, H., Sawtell, M. and Oliver, S. (2005) *Sure Start Plus National Evaluation: Final Report*, London: Social Science Research Unit, Institute of Education, University of London.

Wilkinson, R. (1996) *Unhealthy Societies: The Afflictions of Inequality*, London: Routledge.

Williams, S. J. (1999) 'Is anybody there? Critical realism, chronic illness and the disability debate', *Sociology of Health & Illness*, 21 (6), pp 797-819.

Wilson, N., Syme, S. L., Boyce, W. T., Battistich, V. A. and Selvin, S. (2005) 'Adolescent alcohol, tobacco, and marijuana use: the influence of neighborhood disorder and hope', *American Journal of Health Promotion*, 20 (1), pp 11-19.

Wilson, W. J. (1996) *When Work Disappears*, Chicago, IL: University of Chicago Press.

Wimbush, E., Harper, H., Wright, D., Gruer, L., Lowther, M., Fraser, S. and Gordon, J. (2005) 'Evidence, policy and practice: developing collaborative approaches in Scotland', *Evidence & Policy*, 1 (3), pp 391-407.

Wood, J., Hennell, T., Jones, A., Hooper, J., Tocque, K. and Bellis, M. A. (2006) *Where Wealth Means Health*, Liverpool: North West Public Health Observatory.

Wright, R. (2000) *Nonzero: History, Evolution & Human Cooperation*, London: Abacas.

Wrigley, N., Warm, D. and Margetts, B. (2003) 'Deprivation, diet and food-retail access: findings from the Leeds "food deserts" study', *Environment and Planning A*, 35, pp 151–188.

Wye, C. (2002) *Performance Management: A 'Start Where You Are, Use What You Have' Guide*, Arlington, VA: IBM Endowment for The Business of Government.

Yoh, P. (undated) *Managing Change in Declining Neighbourhoods*, Liverpool: Liverpool City Council.

Zeisel, J., Silverstein, N. M., Hyde, J., Levkoff, S., Lawton, M. P. and Holmes, W. (2003) 'Environmental correlates to behavioral health outcomes in Alzheimer's special care units', *The Gerontologist*, 43, pp 697–711.

Index

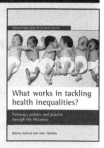
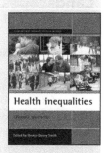

Citizens at the centre
Deliberative participation in healthcare decisions
Celia Davies, Margaret Wetherell and **Elizabeth Barnett**

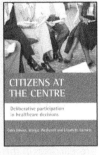

"An engagingly written book that offers a detailed and thoughtful analysis of an innovative experiment in citizen participation in healthcare decision-making. This timely study raises a host of significant challenges for democratic theorists and practitioners alike." **Graham Smith**, Professor of Politics, School of Social Sciences, University of Southampton, UK

Drawing on the lessons from an ethnographic study of a public involvement initiative in the health service, this book sets out to understand what happens when members of the public are drawn into the unfamiliar world of policy making at national level and looks at the contribution that citizens can realistically be expected to make.

Paperback £23.99 US$42.95 ISBN-13 978 1 86134 802 9
Hardback £60.00 US$110.00 ISBN-13 978 1 86134 803 6
234 x 156mm 304 pages October 2006

Landscapes of voluntarism
New spaces of health, welfare and governance
Edited by **Christine Milligan** and **David Conradson**

"Stimulating and informative; this book deals with a broad range of issues (from governance to volunteering) and so provides the reader with a remarkable view of the 'landscape of voluntarism'. There is a wealth of excellent, informed research and this will provide inspiration for students, academics, researchers, practitioners and policy makers alike."
Dr Clare Fisher, Head of Department, Voluntary Sector Studies, University of Wales, Lampeter

Landscapes of Voluntarism explores the complex relationship between voluntary action, society and space. Prefaced by one of the foremost geographers in this field, it explores the interactions between voluntarism and a range of issues including governance, health, community action, faith, ethnicity, counselling, advocacy and professionalisation.

Hardback £55.00 US$75.00 ISBN-13 978 1 86134 632 2
240 x 172mm 320 pages June 2006

Health inequalities and welfare resources
Continuity and change in Sweden
*Edited by **Johan Fritzell** and **Olle Lundberg***

*Foreword by **Lisa Berkman**, Professor of Public Policy, Harvard University*

"The book makes an original and important contribution to the field. It interrogates a rich dataset relating to a society in which there is intense international interest using perspectives at the cutting-edge of health inequalities research." **Hilary Graham**, Professor of Health Sciences, University of York, UK

How welfare states influence population health and health inequalities has long been debated but less well tested by empirical research. This book presents new empirical evidence of the effects of Swedish welfare state structures and policies on the lives of Swedish citizens. The discussion, analysis and innovative theoretical approaches developed in the book have implications for health research and policy beyond Scandinavian borders.

Paperback £24.99 US$39.95 ISBN-13 978 1 86134 757 2
Hardback £55.00 US$90.00 ISBN-13 978 1 86134 758 9
234 x 156mm 256 tbc pages November 2006
Health and Society series

To order copies of this publication or any other Policy Press titles please visit **www.policypress.org.uk** or contact:

In the UK and Europe:
Marston Book Services, PO Box 269, Abingdon, Oxon, OX14 4YN, UK
Tel: +44 (0)1235 465500
Fax: +44 (0)1235 465556
Email:
direct.orders@marston.co.uk

In Australia and New Zealand:
DA Information Services, 648 Whitehorse Road Mitcham, Victoria 3132, Australia
Tel: +61 (3) 9210 7777
Fax: +61 (3) 9210 7788
E-mail:
service@dadirect.com.au

In the USA and Canada:
ISBS, 920 NE 58th Street, Suite 300, Portland, OR 97213-3786, USA
Tel: +1 800 944 6190 (toll free)
Fax: +1 503 280 8832
Email: info@isbs.com

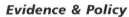
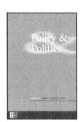

Printed and bound by CPI Group (UK) Ltd, Croydon, CR0 4YY

27/10/2024

14580560-0002